*"Our vision must include looking at every single aspect
of healthcare as an opportunity to innovate,
to create new and better quality services and
products that can be used at home and sold abroad.
That is a tall order."*

Dedication

"To my wife Florence; a great listener and a wonderful friend."

Healthcare

Conflicting Opinions, Tough Decisions

William V. Weiss, MD, CCFP, P. Eng.

NC Press Limited
Toronto, 1992

© William V. Weiss 1992.

No part of this publication may be reproduced, stored in a retrieval system, or transmitted, in any form or by any means, electronic, mechanical, photocopying, recording or otherwise, without the prior written permission of NC Press Limited.

Cover Design: Gerry Ginsberg
Photograph of Dr. Weiss: Claude Noel

Canadian Cataloguing in Publication Data

Weiss, William V., 1938-
  Healthcare

(FAMILYbooks)
Includes bibliographical references and index.
ISBN 1-055021-071-8

I. Medical care - Canada.
2. Medical policy - Canada.   I. Title.   II. Series.
RA449.W45 1992   362.1'0971   C91-095778-9

We would like to thank the Ontario Arts Council, the Ontario Publishing Centre, the Ontario Ministry of Culture and Communications, and the Canada Council for their assistance in the production of this book.

New Canada Publications, a division of NC Press Limited,
Box 452, Station A, Toronto, Ontario, Canada, M5W 1H8.

Printed and bound in Canada

CONTENTS

Acknowledgements   9

Preface   11

Introduction   13

Chapter 1   Health System Crisis: The Paradigm Shift
What's Wrong Depends on Who You Ask   15
Paradigms and Their Relevance to Healthcare   22
A Short History of Medicine: The Placebo Effect and Change   23
The Legacy of National Health Schemes   25
Can the Healthcare Paradigm Shift be Contained   27

Chapter 2   Limitless Patient Demand, Limited Ability to Pay
Temporary Reactions Against the Growing Scope of Medicine   30
The Information Age: The Engine of the Health Paradigm Shift   30
An Evergrowing Industry: The Promise of Youth and Immortality   31
Zero Tolerance: The Consumer Society   35
Fear of Global Environmental Changes: Fueling New Health Services Demand   36
"The Despair of Demographics"   36
Limited Ability to Pay: What Will Medicare Continue to Cover?   38

Chapter 3   Should Canada Consider Going Down the Oregon Trail?
The Oregon Experiment: A Precedent for Others to Follow?   40
The Process: 47 Community Meetings   41
Diagnosis Shift, Specialty Shift   45
Is Rationing Inevitable in Canada?   46

Chapter 4   What Should Medicare Do For Patients
Insurance Against CATASTROPHIC Illness   48
It's No Fun to Say No   50
What Can Modern Medicine Do For Patients?   52
The NIH Consensus Development Program   53
A View From the Other Side: A Previous Ontario Minister of Health Speaks Out   57

Chapter 5   What Should Modern Medicine Do For Patients?
Our Medical Moral Imperative   59
Is the Hospital the Best Place to Deliver Healthcare? It Depends   61

Chapter 6   Motivating the Participants
Why Should Doctors be Forced to Become the Gatekeepers?   66
Cost-Effectiveness Tools in Health Delivery are Not Yet Available   67
Variable Patient Behaviour and Treatment Delays   69
Fiscal Responsibility for Patients   70
Flogging a Dread Public   73
User Fees: Reality Therapy   74
Creating a Market Economy within Medicare   74
The Patient as Gatekeeper?   75
Incentives for Underservicing? No Way!   76

Ideas that Should be Considered	77
Refuse Payment for Sick Notes	80
Pay for Telephone Advice	80
Proposed: A Health-Cost Reduction Motivational Research Organization	81

Chapter 7 Reform, Innovation: Is it Possible, Wanted, or Likely?

Predictable Government Reactions	83
Innovation: Is it Wanted?	85
Provincial Health Ministry Surveillance Systems	87
Unilateral Government Moves	88
Further Barriers to Change and Reform	90
Reform?	93

Chapter 8 What are Our Governments Up To?

Who Should be Going to Emergency?	95
Let Them Use Community Health Centres!	97
Spring's Story	99
Health Service Organizations, Revisited	101
Restricting Out-of-Country Health Plan Payments	103
What Price Consultation? Caps and Clawbacks!	103
Privatization: The Double Standard	105
Do Salaries for Doctors Save Money?	106
Reduce the Numbers of Doctors!	107
Some Twists on the User Fee Theme	108
The Medical Funds Account	109

Chapter 9 Reactions To a Health System in Decline

Brain Drain	111
Alternative Methods of Practice	113
Why Should We Feel Good?	113
Doctor-Bashing	115
Catch-22: High Touch or High Tech?	116
Defensive Medicine	117
Recognition for Excellence	118
Why Most Doctors Don't Want to be on the Payroll	119

Chapter 10 Prevention: The Great Deception?

Does Prevention Save Money?	121
Lack of Energy, Fatigue: A Costly Diagnostic Conundrum	123
Medical Screening/Preventive Medicine: How Can We Pay For It?	126
A Philosophy of Screening from a Physician's Viewpoint	127
Some Unexpected Ramifications of Prevention	128
The Guideline Gap	130
The New Genetics: The Ethical Issues of Knowing	131

Chapter 11 Tough Choices Your Provincial Health Ministry Might Make

Confuse the Public (And Health Professionals)	133
Belt Tightening Under Way as You Read This	133
Blame the Care Providers to Deflect Attention	134
Worst Case Scenario: Privatize All Medical Care Except Catastrophic Care	134

A Gentler Scenario: Make Arbitrary Cuts in Payments, Providers and Services	134
Prevention, Cholesterol and Blood Lipids Revisited	136
HIN Cards and the Smartcard Health Encounter Monitoring Program	138
Monitoring Patient-Provider Service Encounters	141
Shift More Prescription Drugs to Over-the-Counter Status	141
Campaigns to Convince the Public Many Visits to Doctors are Unnecessary	142
Current Services: Eliminated, Limited or Shifted to Less Expensive Personnel	142
Selfcare Encouraged	143
Force All Family Physicians Out of Fee-for-Service and on to Salaries	145

Chapter 12 Health System Waste Management

Some Perspectives on Minimizing Unnecessary Tests	148
Government Waste	149
Quality Assurance	150
Are These Services Wasteful?	150
Does "Managed Care" Make Sense?	150

Chapter 13 High Tech to the Rescue?

Lessons From The Front Line	152
Medical Computing: Why There (Probably) Isn't a Computer...	154
Ontario's Belated Information and Technology Strategic Plan	156
Medical Records and Case Management	157
Telecommunications	159
A National Health Information Utility and Network	159
Canada's Modern Medicine Online (MMOL): A Brief, Unsuccessful Try	161
Optimal Drug Therapy Database	163
Other Services the Health Information Utility Might Provide	164
Medical Mind-net: A First Step	166
Compact Disc Databases (CD-ROM): Possible Staging Tools	167
Interactive Videos: Patients in the Treatment Decision Making Process	167

Chapter 14 The New Economy: Does Canada Want to Participate?

Biotechnology	170
Gene-Splicing to Create Proteins Normally Produced in Humans	171
Biotech Vaccines (Recombinant DNA Technology)	171
Carbohydrate Chemistry	171
Antisense Molecules: Chemicals that Selectively Block Messages in DNA	171
Antibodies	172
Peptide Chemistry	172
Cell Transplant/Gene Therapy	172
Selfcare Using Intelligent Monitoring Devices	173
Enabling Technology Impacting Medical Research and Healthcare	174
Imaging: A Major Trend in Future Health Practices	175
Laser Scanning, Photodynamic Therapy, Confocal Microscopy	177
Molecular Nanotechnology: Molecular Manufacturing	178
Biosensors	179
Clinical Trials: The Engine of Pharmaceutical Change	179

Chapter 15 Why Healthcare Should Be the Biggest Industry on Earth
    We Cannot Afford a Healthcare Monopoly in the Fourth Wave   181
    What We Really Need: Restructuring, Innovation, Market Forces   183
    A Mixture of Public and Private Services   184
    How the Invidual Might Pay for Services Beyond the Universal Medicare Package   185
    Canada Needs a New Health System Vision: A Strategic Plan   187
    The Role of Government   189
    Standards   189
    Quality Assurance   189
    Industrial Strategy   190
    Ways Governments Can Assist Canadian Healthcare Innovations   191
    What Have We Learned From the Old System   193
    Conclusion   195

Appendix A   197

Endnotes   203

Bibliography   206

Index   209

TABLE OF FIGURES

Figure 1	Health and Wealth in OECD Countries OECD Health Care Financing Administration	17
Figure 2	Total Healthcare Spending as % of GDP OECD Health Care Financing Administration	18
Figure 3	The Oregon Plan's Categories of Care Oregon Health Services Commission	42
Figure 4	Healthcare Valuable to Certain Individuals Oregon Health Services Commission	43
Figure 5	Evolution of Technology for Cardiovascular Disease BMJ, Vol. 304, February 1992, p. 497.	46
Figure 6	OECD Health Indicators, 1989 OECD Health Care Financing Administration	51
Figure 7	NIH Consensus Development Program U.S.A. National Institue of Health	54-56
Figure 8	Encounters and Estimated Costs of Doctors Visits in Ontario Ontario Medical Review, January 1992, p. 14.	71

ACKNOWLEDGEMENTS

This book would not have been possible without the encouragement and support of my publisher, Caroline Walker and NC Press. After listening for ten years to my pontificating about the "ills" of the Canadian medical system, and some of my proposed solutions, last summer she challenged me to "put it all down" in a book. Also, much credit and thanks go to Caroline's husband, Norman Endicott, my favourite Counsel, for his advice and for encouraging and questioning my ideas.

I am deeply appreciative of all the time, effort, and advice my wife Florence generously gave to this project. Our endless discussions were invaluable, as were her comments on the manuscript. The past eight months of writing interfered much in our regular routine.

Special thanks go to Elinor Caplan, MPP, for sharing her experience and wisdom gained as Liberal Minister of Health for Ontario. Of particular note are the initiatives undertaken during her administration: the Health Information Number (HIN) Card; and the Information and Technology Strategic Plan, which will help lay the groundwork for many of the data tracking tools I have proposed in this book.

I would like to express my thanks to Tim Lynch, Info-Lynk Consulting, for teaching me much about Canadian health policy and government health care administrative structures. As well, he helped me better understand the pharmaceutical industry and its relations with governments in Canada.

My thanks to consultant Andrew Szonyi, PhD, of Zarex Management. His broad entrepreneurial business experience, in particular his involvement with the Science Council of Canada, and his insights into the machinations of Canadian science policy and long range science planning, were invaluable.

Much gratitude goes to my friend and fellow computer traveler, Don Brady, for his knowledge and teaching in the complexities of software development and telecommunications. He has tremendously enriched my life with his abundant technical skills.

I would also thank the many physicians who put up with my constant questions. In particular, my associate and long-time friend, Dr. Dan Stephen, tirelessly listened and added to my thoughts as they unfolded. My gratitude to Dr. Susan Lenkei-Kerwin, Director, Inpatient Services, Cardiology Division, The Toronto Hospital, for her time and insights in discussing cardiology and related topics in Ontario. Thanks to Dr. Douglas Sanders, Radiologist, The Toronto Hospital, for enlarging my understanding of CT and MRI imaging. As well, much thanks to John Stevens, PhD, also of The Toronto Hospital, for clarifying my confusions about CT, and MRI "volume analysis" and its growing potential in imaging. Thanks to Dr. S. Herschorn, Chief, Division of Urology, Sunnybrook Medical Centre, for his thoughts on Canadian and American urological practices.

Finally, my heartfelt apologies to all my patients who may have felt neglected during the writing of this book. Hopefully things will soon return to normal.

– Dr. Bill Weiss, Toronto, July 1992.

PREFACE

> *To cure sometimes*
> *To relieve often*
> *To comfort, always*
> > Anonymous. From the French, 15th century.

Canada has built a health system we can all be proud of. I am proud of what Canadian medicine has achieved over the years, and I am proud of the continuing efforts of doctors and other healthcare workers to adapt to changing and difficult circumstances. Although we have our troubles currently, so has every other national health system. We must all keep an open mind as we look for new ways to address this challenge.

This book was written in response to the many anxiety-provoking trends in Canada's healthcare environment. Foremost in my mind was the continuing deterioration in morale in health providers and, in spite of occasional successes, in the relations between governments and the medical professions. I am deeply troubled by the philosophy of government that physicians are a commodity to be managed.

While both the public and the health providers can do much more to conserve limited and expensive health resources, there is growing concern among health professionals about the role of cost-containment agent that government wants to place us in. It is far from clear that this is desirable.

In the midst of sweeping and rapid changes in our health system, a very narrow view of what should be done seems to dominate discussion. It is time to take stock of the ways Medicare has evolved and even to reinvent our health system.

The current view is that the Canadian health system or industry must be a government system, alone. Such a narrow view is preventing the entrepreneurial and innovative contributions essential to the continued success of our system. Canada can ill-afford to lose this energy, or worse, drive it elsewhere. Canada's healthcare sector must become more than a sector which "consumes" national wealth. Our health system must become a creator of national wealth. We must not continue to import the vast majority of our health technology from other nations.

Particularly disquieting is how little to date the health system has benefited from the computer and telecommunications revolution. Healthcare is a sector of limitless opportunity for growth in The New Economy, and must not be neglected as Canada restructures its economy for the 21st century.

INTRODUCTION

Canada's Medicare System is under stress. Daily we are exposed to proclamations from television, radio and the print media about its imminent or inevitable collapse. The message grows louder and louder that we are going to have to learn to accept less.[1]

While we Canadians endlessly debate those cultural attributes which identify us uniquely, one of the few things we have been able to find consensus about is our healthcare system, until recently our national pride and joy. Sorting through the howls of despair and the endless commissions and technical documents is difficult for health professionals let alone average citizens. Exactly what is in jeopardy? What is simply media hype? The failing state of our healthcare system has become one of the most popular Canadian topics of conversation, right up there with the daily sports scores, the economy and the likely dissolution of our national union.

There is a great malaise in the healthcare system. A crisis in funding threatens the existence of many hospitals. Workers at every level – hospital presidents, nurses and physicians, ward orderlies – do not have the same good feelings about their jobs that they did in earlier years. Healthcare service, for too many, is not fun any more. Healthcare workers, like many hospitals and health facilities, are somewhat frayed around the edges.

Twenty years ago, the optimistic zeal with which medical interns and nurses began their chosen careers was the fuel that energized the health system. The time from zeal to cynicism was decades. Now it comes during training, as nursing and medical interns see their options shrinking at a blazing rate. Physicians are looking for escape routes to the U.S. or salaried jobs that remove them from direct patient care. Nurses leave the profession for employment in real estate. Why has such previously rewarding work gone sour?

Solving the problem of morale amongst healthcare professionals may be more important than all the funding and administrative initiatives under way to reform the system. Too many health system corporate employees feel pessimistic or apathetic about their mission; we should collectively be looking at solutions which empower these people.

The Canadian healthcare system is stagnating. The lack of competitive spirit in the monopolistic government system is largely responsible for the current situation. Many Canadian healthcare innovators, tired of beating their heads against the massive bureaucratic wall of indifference, have given up trying to change things, turned off or gone to the U.S. Missed opportunities in many areas of our health system have enriched American, European, Japanese, Taiwanese, or Korean companies.

Typical knee-jerk responses to our crisis are:
1. Cap all the doctors' incomes and/or put them all on salary. Initiate stiffer management controls.
2. Close down hospital beds and lay-off some staff.
3. Shrink services.
4. Initiate a Royal Commission to study the problem.

Doctors and nurses are more than a little tired of being blamed for Medicare's success at attracting patients. The fact that healthcare is such an amazingly successful product, and that in any other business this would be good, seems to elude the politicians and administrators. Blaming the purveyors of the best-seller is ludicrous. The blaming just aggravates the participants and inhibits reform. Rarely has any business complained to their customers that their endless demand for the product is a problem!

Throughout the book you will find many references to, and extracts from, current news reports. Much of this book evolved interactively with the media on a daily basis. All the material is thus relevant and timely.

This book is about reinventing Medicare and healthcare in general, about lateral-thinking, innovation, solutions and change. I have tried to put forth some provocative ideas to challenge our complacency. We Canadians have had an historical willingness to allow governments to exert considerable control over our affairs. It is time, I suggest, to look critically at this policy. The state of our economy, and our tardiness in coming to terms with the realities of global competitiveness, are warnings that for too long we have been patting ourselves on the back. Our healthcare system, like our economy, is settling into mediocrity before our eyes.

Expensive warnings from consultants such as Michael Porter, of Harvard, have not led to a renewed national resolve: "We've cut the best trees, mined the best mines, fished the fish, pumped the oil, and made a mint exporting all of it. Now we need a different kind of economy and a host of new export industries to pay the bills."[2] So now what?

Change is uncomfortable. Very few like it, doctor or patient! Without reform, Canadian Medicare will not survive. We will to have to learn to live with shrinking healthcare unless major changes are made to our system. I feel strongly that these are not only desirable, but possible.

CHAPTER 1

HEALTH SYSTEM IN CRISIS: THE PARADIGM SHIFT

We have for years patted ourselves on the back, comparing ourselves to the U.S. We have controlled costs while adhering to the main principles of Medicare: equity, universality, comprehensiveness, accessibility, portability, and non-profit public administration. Meanwhile, the American health systems' costs have been spiraling out of control, while completely excluding upwards of 25% of their population.

What's Wrong Depends on Who You Ask

While there is little consensus amongst the various stakeholders in healthcare as to the cause or the remedy to our current difficulties, everyone seems to agree that the cost of available medical interventions, let alone the numbers of emerging health products and services, exceeds any reasonable fraction of the resources of any developed country.

The restructuring of the Canadian economy, changing demographics, an aging population, rapid technological change, increasingly demanding and knowledgeable consumers, all are driving not only Canada's but every country's health systems into insolvency.

Ask the average Canadian what's wrong and you are likely to get a shrug, since most of us give high ratings to the system and haven't personally experienced a crisis. For most ordinary healthcare encounters with a family doctor, there are minimal delays. Getting appointments with many specialists is becoming more difficult, although the difficulty varies considerably from region to region and community to community. Ophthalmologists (eye doctors) in particular, orthopaedic specialists, and psychiatrists are in short supply. A continuing and as yet unsolved problem is that of Canadians living in the underserviced areas of all provinces. This situation is deteriorating and continues to plague health planners.

There is growing difficulty getting admitted to hospitals, and there is much apprehension about how bad this will get if threatened bed closures occur. Emergency department services are becoming more congested, and people generally expect longer waiting times if they choose this route rather than going to their regular doctors, or to a walk-in clinic for minor problems. The impression is growing that for minor medical problems the Canadian health system is responsive, but for more serious problems, getting the kind of attention we expect is increasingly difficult.

If you were to ask the "Average Canadian" if he or she personally is overutilizing the health system, few would answer in the affirmative. Very few of those taking unusual (excessive) advantage of the system perceive this as being an accurate description of their habits. While people can agree generally about "them out there" they rarely see or admit to any personal fault. Medical professionals and patients have considerably different perceptions about what constitutes appropriate use. Doctors find it almost impossible to challenge patients about over-utilization.

Government officials and politicians at both the national and provincial health funding levels say they firmly believe that nothing fundamental is wrong that cannot be solved by good management and the identification and reduction of the waste. The dimensions of the waste problem currently being tossed around by health system critics is 25-30%. Some believe it is as high as 40-50%! Thus, officials and politicians have come to believe that 25-30% of what is currently being done in the health system is unnecessary and, if eliminated, would solve most of our funding problems. Although doctors continue to be singled out as the principal culprits in all this, there is a growing tendency also to blame hospital administrators and a growing cast of others, including the public.

Provincial health experts have a host of indicators and other statistics to support their arguments that Canadians have more than adequate levels of health service *(Figures 1 and 2)*. We spend twice as much as Great Britain per person (almost $1,800 per year), and are second in the world only to the Americans in annual per capita expenditures ($2,500). Provincial health ministry executives are fond of responding to critics by comparing the successes of Canadian healthcare with the problems of the U.S. health system.

They point out that most of the excesses of the American system are caused by powerful market forces in the over-commercialized medical-industrial complex. Such officials also believe Canadians have an inappropriate concept of what their true health needs are, and that such confusion has been largely caused by poisonous and uncontrollable American health marketing influences/forces leaking across the border. How can a thoughtful Canadian citizen sort out what health needs of a Canadian community are truly appropriate, as opposed to what they are being marketed to believe, by media influences from the U.S.?

The philosophy of the American health system has developed quite differently from ours over the years. It is freewheeling, innovative, technology-intoxicated, entrepreneurial, over-commercialized, competitive and market-driven (consumer-responsive) – and expensive. You can buy all the healthcare you or your boss can afford. Any rationing is by price.

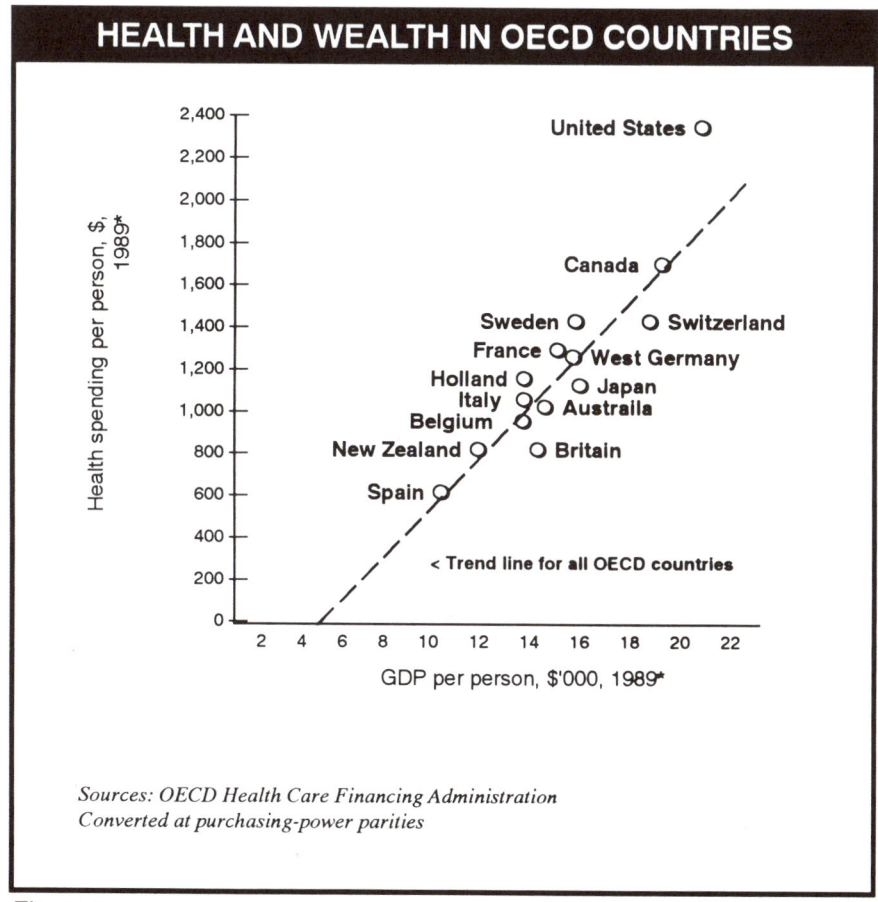

HEALTH AND WEALTH IN OECD COUNTRIES

Health spending per person, $, 1989*
GDP per person, $'000, 1989*

Sources: OECD Health Care Financing Administration
Converted at purchasing-power parities

Figure 1

Healthcare spending as % of GDP

Healthcare spending as % of GDP

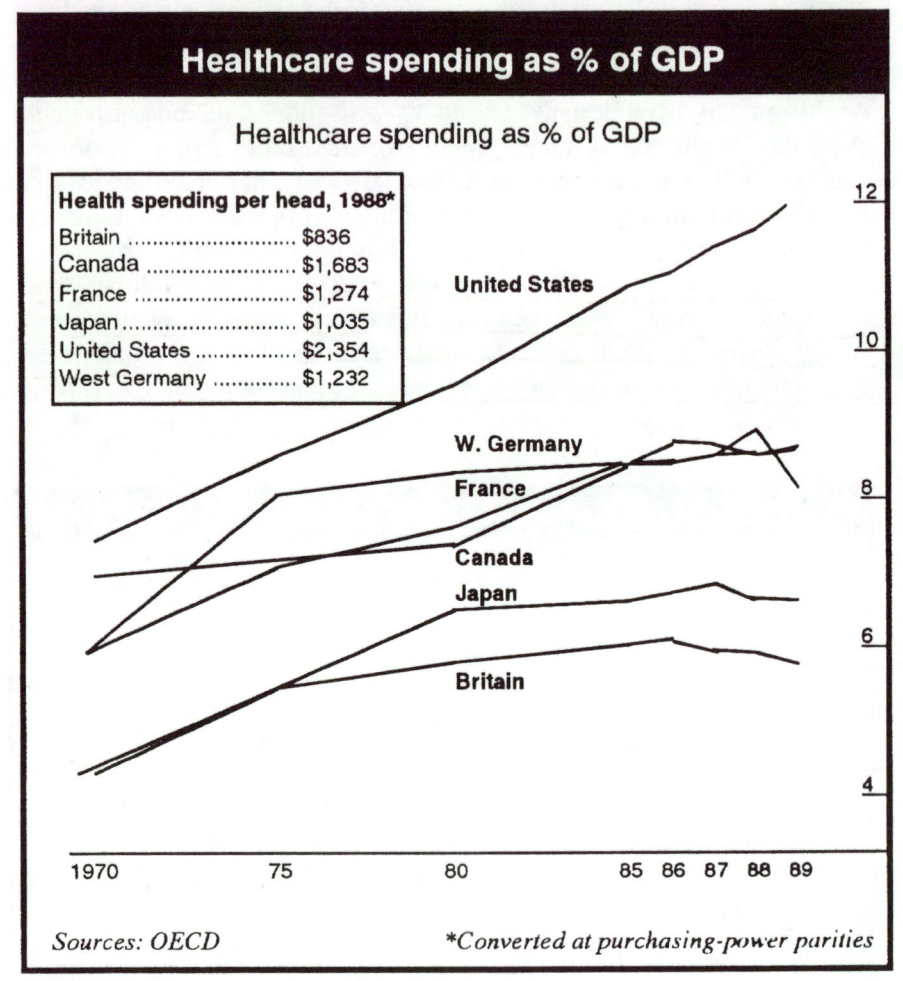

Health spending per head, 1988*

Britain	$836
Canada	$1,683
France	$1,274
Japan	$1,035
United States	$2,354
West Germany	$1,232

Sources: OECD *Converted at purchasing-power parities

Figure 2

Canadian healthcare philosophy is much more conservative and egalitarian. Canadians have a fundamental belief as a nation in equality before the healthcare system. We say, quite simply, that no one ought to be able to buy themselves a better brand of healthcare because they have more money (even though logic and experience suggests this is unenforceable) and that no one should be denied service because they are unable to pay. Thus our system is controlled, relatively rigid, centralized, bureaucratized, and definitely not market-driven. It is nowhere nearly as gadgetized or as commercialized. Any rationing in Canada is far more subtle and concealed. "Envelope funding" of hospitals results in shortfalls of funding being transferred to patients in the form of random reduction of services. Geography imposes regional inequities.

Canadian national television and print media critics well understand that American culture has a major influence on us at many levels, and healthcare is not exempt. Not only does this cultural influence have an effect on Canadian health consumer demand and attitudes, but many American medical and administrative practices influence our government bureaucrats, hospital executives and medical professionals.

Asking doctors what is wrong is confusing because they have no consensus on the subject. Every specialty has opinions. Most doctors are very defensive about the issue of wasteful medical interventions, and their part in it. Collectively, doctors admit to some wasteful practices, but they tend to defend them as a response to patient or consumer demand, or their concern about litigation. They also argue that wasteful or ineffectual practices are too expensive difficult, and time consuming to identify completely. Most doctors would argue that it is extremely naive of governments to believe that, even if we could identify and eliminate significant amounts of wasteful practice, this would solve Medicare's financial problems for the long term.

Generally the hospital-based specialists believe the family practitioners do too many tests and account for more health system waste than they do. For their part, the family practitioners believe the academic and training-based doctors do too many tests in their treatment of patients. Perhaps the government can tell us the correct answer to this one? Most primary care physicians (primarily family doctors) believe procedure-oriented specialists earn excessive amounts for doing high technology procedures, compared to cognitive or non-procedure-oriented physicians. Generally, however, people agree that it is these high technology procedures (and the specialists who perform them) that should command the highest fees. This public attitude drives the cost of healthcare ever upwards.

Both doctors and nurses generally agree that Canada's Right to Health has created and continues to create unbelievable, unconscionable and frequent abuse of the system. Several interesting anecdotes might demonstrate their frustrations, not with the stereotypical "abuser" but with you and me.

A friend of ours recently spent a day in hospital to undergo a breast biopsy (the surgeon removes a piece of tissue for microscopic pathology examination). She relayed these anecdotes to my wife. After her biopsy, in the recovery room, she overheard two nurses complaining to each other about the waste caused by one of the day's patients. Apparently a woman, who had previously had a tubal ligation to prevent further pregnancies, had changed her mind and was in hospital to have the procedure reversed. The nurses agreed that the taxpayers should not have to bear this expense. They were clearly frustrated because the healthcare system is being blamed for rising costs, when in reality, patient demand is a critical factor.

Her second story involved her pre-surgery tests, which included a chest X-ray. As she was being prepared for the X-ray, our friend mentioned that she had concerns over too much radiation, since she had had a chest X-ray a few months earlier. The technician then berated our friend, explaining that this was why health costs kept spiraling. She was asked why she didn't just have these recent X-rays sent to the hospital. Of course she hadn't thought of it and had never been asked. She readily accepted the chastisement, which she felt legitimate . . . she did wonder, however, why no one (her doctor?) had even attempted to coordinate all these aspects of her treatment.

"My answer to the valid concern re redundant tests," many doctors would simply reply, "is that it is easier to order them again at our own laboratory than to try and 'extract' a report or test from some other facility." As well, some doctors feel tests ordered at their facility are more reliable than those from elsewhere! And so it goes.

So, what does this illustrate? Poor communication by healthcare professionals leading to duplication. What else is new? Many patients tell me that they have had to return for blood tests several times (and experience the pain of two needle punctures), because the entire set of tests on my lab requisition was not completed, somehow missed or neglected by the technician. Other than apologizing, I never know how to answer such complaints. This kind of waste occurs at every level and, aside from allowing everyone the occasional mistake, it is inexcusable.

One last glaring example of Medicare money wastage occurs at the pharmacy counter. In Ontario and other provinces, seniors (over 65) and persons on welfare receive their prescriptions free. A commonly prescribed drug is Aspirin or simple acetylsalicylic acid (ASA). Many doctors are properly prescribing ASA for many of these patients, in modest doses (325 mg or less per day), as a preventive platelet inhibiting agent or "blood thinner" for heart attack and stroke prevention. Whether "enteric-coated" or plain, ASA tablets cost the pharmacy pennies per pill. And yet the pharmacy, when it fills that prescription for ASA (which in total might be less than a dollar), charges Medicare eight dollars for the service!

If the vast numbers of patients currently receiving JUST ASA were to pay out-of-pocket for their ASA and buy it over the counter, and even be reimbursed later, it could save the system millions and perhaps tens of millions of dollars for this item alone. There are many other examples of inexpensive prescription and non-prescription drugs.

If the diverse specialties of medicine can agree on anything, they would all probably agree that growing fear of malpractice litigation, and patient attitudes and expectations of what modern medicine should deliver, are a common source of anxiety, frustration, and defensive medical practices. Such practices result in costly over-investigation of patients, so as to avoid missing anything.

But physicians are far more concerned about deteriorating morale at every level in the health system. Many Canadian medical specialists receive their post-graduate medical training in the U.S. and thus have a desire to use the same technologies and techniques locally that they employed during their residency. As well, many Canadian doctors attend continuing medical education conferences in the U.S. and thus are acquainted with the tools and techniques their American colleagues are using. Finally, most Canadian doctors regularly receive medical journals from the U.S. All of these sources keep their interest in American technologies high enough to influence their attitudes and practices in Canada.

What has all this to do with what Canadian doctors believe is wrong with our system? Many believe we are falling behind in the application of appropriate technologies. Some of our best specialists are leaving for the U.S. because they can't get the tools or operating room time they need in Canada to do their job for their patients as they would like to do it.

Ask hospital administrators what is wrong and they tend to believe that they are under-funded, that employee salaries are too high, that they are over-regulated, patient loads are excessive, and that facilities are suffering from the effects of age and insufficient maintenance. Many administrators feel constrained in their freedom to react to market opportunities, make decisions, and that provincial health ministries respond too slowly to their requests and concerns. Many feel they lack access to certain diagnostic procedures, like Magnetic Resonance Imaging (MRI). Most would like to implement better management information systems but lack resources to do so.

Until recently it was not uncommon for hospitals to request and receive annual increases in budgets of more than ten percent. For years it was almost an article of faith that increased costs could simply be passed on to government for more money. In spite of warnings by most provincial health ministries that such increases could not continue, few hospitals actively prepared for the current freeze. A combination of a poor and declining Canadian economy, an aging population, annual increases in patient demand and doctors' services, rapid technological change and, finally, a federal government decision starting in 1985 to reduce health transfer payments to the provinces, dealt a knockout punch to provincial health economics.

We all knew some time back that uncontrolled growth in health services could not continue indefinitely, but this did not seem to motivate us, individually or collectively, to take measures to reduce system usage and wasteful practices. For many years, physician services delivered in the fee-for-service side of practice (over 75% of all doctors) have been increasing almost 15% annually. There were never any incentives for the public or doctors to reduce utilization, to change direction. Our current system, in fact, rewards profligacy, not parsimony.

Paradigms and Their Relevance to Healthcare

The dictionary defines a paradigm as an example, pattern or model. A better definition of this term is "a set of rules or regulations about how a concept is perceived." As we grow and learn about the world, we employ many paradigms. But paradigms can change. When they do, it is very difficult (in most cases actually impossible) for people to perceive or understand the subtleties of that change, so steeped do we become in the status quo.

Let me give an example. In 1967, Switzerland was the world leader in wrist-watch, pocket-watch and other clock manufacturing. The Swiss had about 70% of the world market in timepieces, and had dominated it for over a hundred years. Then someone invented the quartz clock. This simple electronic device offered tremendous gains in timing accuracy at much less cost. Two companies, Texas Instruments in the USA and Seiko in Japan, picked up on this technological innovation, and started manufacturing timepieces (primarily watches) based on this new technology. Within a decade the Swiss had lost almost their entire market share of the watch industry. Switzerland lost over 50,000 jobs and the industry was almost bankrupted. It did not matter what their previous experience or expertise had been. The rules had been rewritten; a paradigm shift had occurred.

When the rules are rewritten, everyone goes back to square one or ground zero. Previous position in the market and experience do not matter. The Swiss did not recognize how important the quartz clock innovation was! They were so blinded by the old paradigm of mechanical timepiece design and manufacturing that they could not perceive the implications of this innovation and its impact on their world. What is even more startling was that the quartz clock was invented by Swiss technologists! The Swiss were so confident of their control of this industry that they did not even patent the quartz clock, and placed it in the public domain. Others recognized its immense potential and nearly killed the Swiss watch industry.

What does the concept of paradigm shift have to do with healthcare? Very much more than you can imagine. Medicine and healthcare are in the midst of a paradigm shift; the rules are being rewritten. A crucial change is underway, and to date, there appears to be little understanding of the catastrophic ramifications it will have for all health systems. It is imperative that both the public and government recognize this critical fact. If we do not understand this, we will make incorrect and costly blunders in our attempts at coping with change.

A Short History of Medicine: The Placebo Effect and Change

Let's go back and briefly review the history of medicine. In all history up to modern times, medicine or healing was performed by unscientific practitioners or healers, who learned their art in a piecemeal fashion at the feet of previous practitioners or shamans. They practiced their art on a one-on-one basis with patients. No one really knew much about what they were doing.

Much of the art and success of the healer (then and now) is recognized by most scientists as having been a result of the placebo effect. The placebo effect is the positive reaction a patient experiences from healing, caring, attention, whether it comes from priest, minister, rabbi, shaman, doctor, nurse or other caring and concerned person/s. It is a complex and still poorly understood phenomenon, but it has been one of the most important aspects of care for millennia. Suggestion plays an important role in the placebo effect, and in the context within which the effect occurs. If people believe in the power of a person, or their art (tools, herbs, potions, etc.), then a self-fulfilling healing power is associated with their practices.

A powerful example of the healing power of the mind and our expectations was recently described by Leonard Sagan, in his book *The Health of Nations* (1987). He describes an extraordinary phenomenon noted in many poor Third World countries which seems to fly in the face of most medical science. It had been noted that children in these nations suffering from simple childhood infections such as chicken pox, mumps, or measles, had a mortality rate 200 times higher than in North America. In order to understand this more clearly, a child population was carefully chosen in which all the normal public health measures were in effect. Vaccinations were similar to North American, water supply was clean and uncontaminated, diet was reasonable, etc. Sure enough, the children still died at an incredibly high rate.

The only conclusion the researchers, and the author Leonard Sagan, could come up with to explain the difference between this population and industrialized children was chronic hopelessness and despair. Chronic hopelessness and despair seem to impair the immune systems of these Third World children so they cannot fight off infections which do not even faze kids from happier environments. This is an hypothesis only, but we all know how such powerful emotions can effect the outlook and even the survival of, for example, cancer patients.

Back to medicine's evolution. In addition to the placebo effect, some therapeutic lore gradually developed into a smattering of anecdotal experience using natural plants, potions derived from plants, and so on. We now recognize that the pharmacology of plants is very complex, and there are many new drugs yet to be discovered in the diminishing tropical forests of the world. Not only did ancient man have some knowledge of these plants, but there is recent evidence that even chimpanzees in the wild use plants for medicinal purposes, mostly to rid themselves of intestinal parasites! It may be that that is precisely how man first got the ideas which evolved into herbal medicine. However, there was little true scientific understanding or basis in any of this until very late in the 18th century. The term "healthcare" is derived from the plain and simple fact that caring was about the only thing healers and nurses could offer their patients in the past.

Over the ages there is scattered evidence that a few cultures understood that certain surgical procedures could have dramatic positive effects on the outcomes of certain emergencies, but there was little scientific understanding underlying them. Only with the advent of modern anesthesia could surgery be performed painlessly and more or less reliably, and this was very recent (late 19th century) in the long march of medical history. With the advent of reliable and safe anesthesia, the rapid progress of surgery began.

Only with the rise of the scientific method, with its critical demand for observable facts and reproducible experiments, did the theoretical and scientific basis of disease and its treatment emerge. Before this it was mostly hocus-pocus, magic, a bit of herbalism, and the very important placebo effect.

Only at the end of the Second World War did powerful antibiotics emerge, and they were not available in any volume until the early Fifties. The modern pharmaceutical industry really started to take off after this development. There had been pharmaceutical manufacturers, but they were small in comparison to the global industrial giants that have emerged as modern science began unlocking the secrets about how chemistry, biochemistry, immunology, genetics and physiology interact. So the old helplessness of the care-givers gradually gave way to scientifically-based healthcare which could deliver much more than simple human concern and attention and the placebo effect.

With the advent of modern understanding of the role of public health measures in reducing infectious disease, the use of vaccines to prevent most of the previously lethal infectious diseases, and the medical use of antibiotics to prevent infections from wreaking their historical havoc on populations, modern medicine started to take off as an economic power in national economies. Then, modern medical science started to focus powerful scientific attention on the other infirmities which are responsible for the chronic diseases of mankind: cancer, atherosclerosis and associated vascular and heart disease, arthritis, neurodegenerative diseases, immunological diseases, etc. The costs of applying the scientific method to all aspects of illness and biology were to become so high that insurance and Medicare schemes would be required for ordinary people to afford such care.

The Legacy of National Health Schemes

In the late Forties, Britain and other countries began to develop national health schemes to make available to all their citizens the limited and very early (compared to today and tomorrow) achievements of scientifically-based medicine. Medicare schemes were based on the principle that catastrophic illness could be prevented from economically destroying a family if modern medicine, with its increasingly complex hospitals and specialized professionals, was freely accessible by all patients in time of need. Somehow, however, gradually, ALL the interventions that modern medical science was explosively creating came under the ever-enlarging umbrella of healthcare coverage.

It is my contention that the well-meaning intention of universality that Medicare attempted to address forty years ago, was grounded in an old paradigm of healthcare. A limited, finite and expensive number of interventions were available which, if made available to citizens in time of need, could prevent catastrophic illness from impoverishing a family and return (in many cases) the patient to a productive life after recovery. The advances that would occur in the intervening three decades were inconceivable at the inception of Medicare. The advances that occurred in the past one or two decades will pale in comparison to the future rate of increase of availability of new health services.

As well, in the old health system you only went to the doctor when you had particular kinds of symptoms, or your symptoms had become so severe as to no longer be ignored. Today, and tomorrow, is the era of going to doctors when you have no symptoms! You go to be reassured everything is okay at the moment. Soon, you will go to be reassured everything will be all right in the future! Thus, we are leaving the era of symptomatic medicine and entering into the era of what we doctors call asymptomatic or subclinical medicine.

In such an environment, we can only reassure people that everything is okay if all their costly tests are okay, since they have no physical complaints! Simple current examples of medical problems that have no symptoms (at early and intermediate stages) include diabetes, high blood pressure, high blood cholesterol, early coronary artery narrowing, early abdominal aneurysm, slowly degenerating cartilage in joints, osteoporosis (thinning bones), and very early cancer. Simply doing all the right personal preventive things will certainly help minimize some of these problems, but it won't eliminate all of them! Tomorrow (very soon) people will be routinely having complex panels of genetic screening tests.

No modern Medicare system has understood the implications of the media and of consumerism in the commoditization of health services. Finally, and even more dangerous, no modern health system has taken into account the impact of the revolutionary changes being fueled by technology and molecular biology, in the context of "The Age of Information."[1]

An infinite number of medical interventions are pouring out of an exploding number of biological research laboratories. Every complex tool of modern high technology, from every scientific discipline, is being focused on unraveling the mysteries of cancer, the human brain, and the human genetic code.

This expanding research will not only address solutions to catastrophic illness, but will impact on every conceivable aspect of human biology, at every age level. No aspect of human, animal or even plant existence will remain untouched by these advances. These advances are happening far more rapidly than anyone could have predicted. Mankind has reached the very threshold of dramatically and quickly altering its four billion years of biological evolutionary history. **Mankind will, in fact, now begin to alter its future genetic evolution by design.**

Governments must realize that no health plan, Medicare, private medical insurance, or a combination thereof, will be able to pay for all the products and services on the way, and philosophically they should not be trying to do so. The scope of modern medicine and biological science has far outstripped any of the old healthcare paradigms. Healthcare is no longer one thing but many things. It is no longer a single industry but many industries. Very soon it will be many more industries. It is not capable of being contained by the old paradigm any longer.

Can the Healthcare Paradigm Shift be Contained?

No, it has developed a life of its own. To complicate this further, we are seeing a profound transformation in the way scientists view the physical world. We are shifting from the past three centuries of a mechanistic (atoms, particles) or materialistic view of matter, to a post-mechanistic paradigm.[2] In this view of reality, non-linear and chaotic behaviour models will supersede the older linear methods. New theories will be required to explain and describe the self-organizing principles which led to life itself. Physics and biology will come together in a holistic view of the universe (as opposed to a reductionist view) and all its components. In this environment, the role of ideas and information supersede the production of commodities.

The current atmosphere, in which economists view the entire health and biotechnology industry as one of the most promising and vital for the next several decades or longer (The New Economy), and the limitless awe and fascination with which biological and health sciences are held by the public, just speed up the shift. We developed the attitude that there is, or should be, a cure for any health problem. Our perception of what medicine can do for us will increasingly continue to exceed the actual state of the art. Unsatisfactory medical interventions are becoming less and less acceptable.

Can the paradigm shift be stopped? Not in this post-industrial Age of Information. As long as the public retains this interest in things medical, and R & D planners believe health insurers, government, and the public will pay for advances in health technologies, the momentum currently heating up the molecular biology revolution cannot be held in check. Nothing short of total collapse of our political and economic systems and a return to the Dark Ages will put brakes on the coming change.

Three or four decades ago, you could barely drag most citizens to a doctor or a hospital. Hospitals were a place where people went to die! People feared doctors and healers. Most people well understood how poor their odds were. It took all the intervening years to gradually convince the public that it was relatively safe to seek medical attention (iatrogenic illness proponents would still argue against this presumption). Now most North Americans are plainly enamoured of medical science's increasing victories over time and nature, and have growing confidence in the future potential of the current research activity. This is part of the paradigm shift from forced usage of health care (by emergency circumstances), to regular use of health services as commodities. According to Tom Peters, a well-known American management guru and author of *In Search of Excellence, A Passion for Excellence* and *Thriving on Chaos*, ALL goods and services are en route to becoming commodities.

Governments can try to downsize hospitals, decentralize care from doctors to community clinics, put doctors on salary, shift health care delivery from doctors to allied health personnel, measure and scrutinize all aspects of the health system, but that is not going to contain the paradigm shift.

CHAPTER 2

LIMITLESS PATIENT DEMAND, LIMITED ABILITY TO PAY

When the British National Health Service (NHS) was initiated by Lord Beveridge shortly after the Second World War, it was based on the assumption that there exists in every population a strictly limited amount of morbidity (ill-health) which, if treated under conditions of equity, will eventually decline. Beveridge and his welfare economists naively believed the annual cost of the Health Service would actually fall as this fixed pool (backlog) of illness was cleared away!

The planners and welfare economists did not anticipate that the National Health Service and the public's gradual redefinition of health would broaden the scope of medical care until only budgetary restrictions would keep it from expanding indefinitely. They did not anticipate the impact of the Information Age and consumerism. They did not anticipate a paradigm shift to a consumerist commodity health system. This is the NHS legacy with which all nations are currently struggling.

Canada put in place a similar centralized Medicare system in 1971, leaving out (as did all national health systems) the most important force for moderation: built-in incentives on the part of patients and health service providers to minimize costs by the rational method of economic self-denial (individual fiscal responsibility) operative in every other sphere of life.

As most observers have noted, the Eighties was an era of greed and excess. This decade spawned the collapse of financial empires and institutions, finally culminating in the destruction of many U.S. Savings and Loan institutions, and the jailing of Ivan Boesky, perhaps the model for Gordon Gecko as portrayed by Michael Douglas in the popular movie, *Wall Street*. Should we be surprised that greed in the world of business would spill over into the healthcare system?

The message from the government until very recently was "the healthcare dinner table is set, come and get it" and the public haven't stopped coming. Fueled by tantalizing television programs, articles in the media about medical technology's relentless generation of new products and services, the shopping lists patients arrive with are sometimes truly outrageous.

Temporary Reactions Against the Growing Scope of Medicine

The usual scapegoats are the overpaid, self-serving doctors. Ivan Illich, in his book *Limits To Medicine* (1976), railed against the growing dangers of the medical-industrial complex. He warned of the danger of the medical profession's relentless "medicalization" of everything from birth to existential distress and death. He warned of the growing dangers of iatrogenesis (doctor-inflicted illness). He warned that medicine is interfering with people's ability to cope with natural stages of life. He wrote: "People need no bureaucratic interference to mate, give birth, share the human condition and die. Man's consciously lived fragility, individuality and relatedness make the experience of pain, of sickness and of death, an integral part of his life. The ability to cope with this trio autonomously is fundamental to his health."

Based on our collective global experience of almost half a century of socialized medicine, one might think we should now have some more innovative ideas on how to reform and improve the system. Little such insight appears to be forthcoming. Most of the current writing has been long on who's to blame, and short on what to do about it.

The Information Age: The Engine of the Health Paradigm Shift

Is it likely or even realistic to expect the public to reduce their demands on the healthcare system? Will we heed government calls to eliminate frivolous, "wasteful" or inappropriate medical encounters? Not a chance! In fact, an ever growing number of economists are now regularly predicting that the healthcare, telecommunications, and computer information sectors are the most promising growth areas globally in what they now describe as "The New Economy." Will physicians reduce utilization by denying patients service? Not likely without being legislated by government to do so. Barring economic disincentives or Draconian control measures to moderate demand, the rapidly growing list of health goodies is just too appealing to the public and to doctors.

Our society is obsessed with health. Almost every Canadian television network and local station is now running regular health programs. To name only a few regulars: TV Ontario's "Lifelines" and "Vital Signs," and a new CBC program, "The Medicine File," not to mention "Healthline" on radio. Add these to regular offerings such as "Vista" and "Nova" from the U.S. networks and Public Broadcasting System channels, and the public is invited to become intoxicated with the marvels of modern medical science. This "health science entertainment" does not include the growing role of print media, newspaper and magazine articles, in stimulating the collective health appetite. Most newspapers have a daily or weekly "Medical Watch" or "What's New in Health?" column. It is becoming more and more common for patients to bring in newspaper clippings or magazine articles just to make certain their doctor is aware of the latest information on their specific problem/s.

This news and documentary reporting does not include the powerful role of entertainment programming, in television and film, further fueling unrealistic, even distorted public perceptions of the power of medicine. "The Six Million Dollar Man," and other science fiction medical dramas, are changing the public's perception of modern medicine. Movies such as *The Terminator*, *Robocop*, the *Star Trek* series, *Blade Runner*, *The Adromeda Strain*, *Coma*, and *Terminal Man* all, increasingly, feed the public's imagination with an unrealistic, even surrealistic view of what modern medicine can currently achieve.

An Evergrowing Industry: The Promise of Youth and Immortality

A popular U.S. magazine, *Longevity*, is prototypical of the burgeoning popularized health communications promising optimal youthfulness, delayed aging and extended life, if the reader follows editorial advice and utilizes all the appropriate pharmaceutical potions. Many of these goodies are prescription drugs and require physician intervention. There was never a time when the quest for the elusive fountain of youth has attracted so many.

Each issue contains bulletins hailing the latest advances. No one needs to be reminded about the lightning speed with which steroid abuse spread among the iron pumping and competitive athlete set. Recently Human Growth Hormone has attracted growing attention from performance athletes and in the lucrative longevity market. This drug was originally intended for treatment of those very few children, with a defect in its natural production, who were previously doomed to lifelong dwarfism. This expensive drug ($9000+ for one year) reverses childhood growth hormone deficiency and its effects, and is only one of the new recombinant DNA marvels from pharmaceutical molecular biologists. There is growing evidence that Human Growth Hormone may reverse or impede the havoc wreaked by normal aging processes. Rumours abound that Olympic athletes are using it.

Next came Deprenyl. Deprenyl (seligilene) was recently approved by both the Canadian Health Protection Branch (HPB), and the U.S. Federal Drug Administration (FDA) for use by patients with Parkinson's Disease. However, soon after its release for Parkinson's Disease, rumours started by its promoters began circulating in the press that it enhances longevity if one begins taking it in one's forties and continues for the rest of one's life. These rumours are fueled by animal research underway in the U.S. at a subsidiary of Deprenyl Research Limited, Deprenyl Animal Research, regarding its effect on the longevity of dogs. There is interest in similar trials with cats, and if both are promising, applications to the authorities for permission to incorporate seligilene in cat and dog food products will follow. Most of these unofficial uses of controlled drugs are as yet unconfirmed by scientific tests, but that never appears to lower interest in their illicit use. After all, try and convince a young athlete that steroids are bad for him/her!

Dr. Morton Shulman, CEO of Deprenyl Research, was briefly interviewed, and mention was made of Alzene, one of Deprenyl's new drugs which is undergoing clinical trials for Alzheimer's Disease and other neurodegenerative conditions. This is only one of over a hundred investigational drugs under development by a number of pharmaceutical companies in the cognitive enhancement area.

It is still too early to know whether any of this research will bear fruit, but many doctors believe that true cognitive enhancement drugs will emerge in the next ten years.

The February 1992 issue of *Longevity* includes a long article about the work cellular biologist Michael West is doing at the University of Texas Southwestern Medical Centre in Dallas. West believes that he and his colleagues have identified the genes that not only participate in cellular aging but also play a major role in two of the biggest killers – heart disease and stroke – as well as Alzheimer's Disease. If that isn't enough, West claims he has identified a substance, "senstatin," that utterly destroys the power of these genes. He believes senstatin may help reverse these conditions and may extend human longevity. Sound good? West has excellent scientific credentials, and some take him quite seriously.

On a recent TV Ontario "Market Watch" program, the topic of "smart drugs" was explored. They interviewed John Morgenthaler, co-author of a recent book, *Smart Drugs and Nutrients*, a kind of handbook for cognitive enhancers. The author tries to make the point in his book that whereas most doctors don't believe much in this currently, he believes cognitive performance enhancement is as much a legitimate use of drugs as is the treatment of disease.

In the interview, Morgenthaler mentioned the use of a very old drug, Hydergine, which is supposed to improve cerebral circulation, as one of the mental function enhancers young people are using. This drug is only available by prescription, and has been prescribed in the past to senile patients in an attempt to improve mental functioning. Most doctors do not believe it has any effect and it has fallen out of use.

The most astonishing example recently of elite athletes putting their lives at risk in order to win is the recombinant erythropoietin (rEPO) story. Nineteen European cyclists have died in the past four years most probably as a result of taking this drug. "They often died days after a race," according to Dr. Randy Eichner of the University of Oklahoma Heath Science Centre, at the recent 37th Annual Meeting of the American College of Sports Medicine. "All were under 32 years of age." Neither Eichner nor others looking into this rash of sudden deaths have absolutely confirmed that rEPO was the cause. The deaths of 14 Dutch and five Belgian cyclists began early in 1987, months after the introduction of rEPO. Dutch and Belgian authorities still attribute them to acute myocarditis (an inflammatory destruction of heart muscle, not well understood), although they were unwilling to release autopsy reports to support this diagnosis.

rEPO is the synthetic form of the naturally-produced hormone erythropoietin (EPO), a growth factor which stimulates the bone marrow to produce red blood cells. Its primary medical use to date is for anaemic kidney patients who are unable to produce enough EPO. Since it became available in 1986, rEPO has eliminated the need for transfusions among many dialysis and other types of patients. Recently it has been used to treat AIDS patients receiving AZT.

In normal healthy individuals treated with rEPO, the marrow produces a greater than normal number of erythrocytes (red blood cells). After a series of rEPO injections, a normal haematocrit of 40 may shoot up to 70. The danger is that blood thickens as the concentration of erythrocytes rises. In haematocrits between 60 and 70, the viscosity of the blood may double, and systolic blood pressure soars, sometimes exceeding 210 in young athletes (normal systolic blood pressure during exercise is 150-180). Intense sweating during competition further concentrates the blood. Eventually the blood turns to "mud" and death ensues. Rumours abound that runners are now starting to use this potentially lethal drug. Dr. Peter Snell of the University of Texas Southwestern Medical Center has called for testing of all competitive cyclists, runners and pentatheletes. Any athlete with a haematocrit of over 50, he thinks, should be banned.

This fascination with modern pharmacology, fanned by the media, is just the thin edge of the wedge, as the public becomes ever more knowledgeable about potential benefits of new discoveries. The number of new growth factors mentioned above, now available and still emerging from the labs, capable of stimulating just about every type of cell in the human body to exceed normal levels of function, are frightening to contemplate. Currently, 18 growth factors have been identified and produced synthetically using recombinant DNA technology. Two of these have been released by the FDA for regular use in patient care. Others are currently in clinical trials and more are expected momentarily.

This global fascination (obsession) with health matters, which is part of the paradigm shift and which is most highly developed in North America, has created a phenomenon which has recently begun to complicate normal scientific publishing of medical treatment results. So many print and television journalists currently earn their livelihood tracking technological advances in scientific fields that often consumers know more about specific health advances than their health professionals do! In fact, a popular column, "What Your Patients Are Reading," in *The Medical Post*, a Canadian medical tabloid published by McLean-Hunter, Monica Shea provides abstracts from recent medical articles or original articles appearing in popular magazines. Often, items in these magazines are the only information a doctor might have of some current medical advances, if patients had not informed him/her about it. These articles are in effect a new marketing vehicle for companies promoting new health products.

There is a problem created when journalists report about incomplete and ongoing scientific research and its highly tentative conclusions. It can result in the unrealistically raised expectations of the public and in confusion for doctors. This trend can only be expected to escalate in coming years.

An even more fascinating development, still much less common than the public consumption of daily health news, is the growth of popular medical or health special interest groups on telecommunication networks across North America. On Compuserve, Prodigy, Dialog, and a host of Bulletin Board Systems or BBSs, can be found not only one, but often many different health subject "chat" groups to which anyone with a office or home computer, a modem and a telephone, can dial up and find out the latest information about almost any specific illness. Physicians as a group are far behind knowledgeable consumers in using such information databases.

Self-help and non-profit medical organizations are keeping members informed of the latest treatments in their special interest area. Thus, people suffering from cancer, migraine, heart disease, cystic fibrosis, Lupus, ALS, Parkinson's, Alzheimer's, multiple sclerosis, colitis, muscular dystrophy, diabetes, to name only a few groups, can keep current. These support organizations contribute not only as excellent supplemental resources for their members, but they whet appetites for a cure or remedy just around the corner.

The demand resulting from patients' exposure to private and public access information will explode in the next several years. Any bureaucrat hoping to control such burgeoning healthcare demand might better find another type of employment. It is simply unstoppable! It would take the entire national health budget spent on countering the current media's driving of this demand, just to make a dent in public misperception of the role or appropriateness of healthcare services.

Zero Tolerance: The Consumer Society

We have just described how the media and the information revolution have forever changed public notions of what the health system can do for them. But the story doesn't end here. It is far more complex and malignant. If information excess has whetted appetites for medical interventions, think for a moment about the influences of the Consumer Society on public attitudes?

A generation ago, most people would accept anything the medical profession could do for them with thanks and admiration, the good and the bad news. If Mom or Dad were found to have a terminal illness, we accepted with equanimity. If a baby died at birth, it was God's will. Today, anything short of a perfect outcome raises suspicions of incompetence, and blame must be assigned to someone or some institution.

It has come to pass that more and more people are developing zero tolerance for imperfect outcomes. It is almost as though the goal of zero defect manufacturing perfection pioneered by Japanese industries must become the accepted level of practice in healthcare delivery. The North American legal system, as well as consumerism, bears part of the responsibility for this uncomfortable and unrealistic state of affairs.

North American attitudes about what to expect from the health system are exaggerated and unrealistic. This growing sense of health entitlement is interfering with the system's ability to function. Recently Peter Jennings, on U.S. network television, had a short piece about the American health system crisis. He identified the American public's attitude about what the health system should deliver as the over-riding challenge to reform. People want the best. People want someone else to pay, and they don't care too much who, as long as it is not them. There is no awareness of cost and little concern other than that they get the best. Medicine can fix anything. Death is the result of mistakes or a lack of the proper tools.

Fear of Global Environmental Changes: Fueling New Health Services Demands

We have already noted irreversible forces increasing health system utilization. We have not yet begun to tap the universal fear that environmental collapse is engendering: "Holes in the Ozone Layer," "Global Warming," "Red Tides." The news recently has been filled with alarms about the ramifications of these changes. The loss of protection from solar ultra-violet light (UV), caused by increasing loss of the ozone layer, has recognized human and plant effects: increased skin cancers and other cancers, and reduced immunological resistance.

People are already seeking medical attention for a host of related or unrelated symptoms which they believe might be related to these changing environmental conditions. They are demanding reassurance that their "immune functions" are normal, even in the absence of present objective medical methods to actually do this.

"The Despair of the Demographics"

By the year 2020, over six million Canadian will be over 65, twice as many as today – one in five. In 1989, our seniors (only 11.3% of the population) accounted for over 40% of healthcare expenditures. Life expectancy is increasing, for women especially, and those over 75 years of age took up more than one-third of all hospital days in 1989. Citizens over 65 use 44% of drug benefits in Saskatchewan's universal drug benefit plan. These statistics are the most frightening and most inexorable indicators of future demands on our health system.[1]

The usual response for the experts and ideologues is to point out that the elderly in Canada are over-doctored, over-medicated and over-hospitalized. All this is undoubtedly true, but who is to take the political rap for deciding when the elderly should see a doctor, which drugs are to be provided free to seniors, and when your Aunt Jane is to be put into hospital and what hospital? And, by the way, when is her treatment to be curtailed?

No government or group has stepped forward to take the lead in solving the massive problems that are fast overtaking us. However, there is a frightening tendency to attack the problem piecemeal:

- *Making euthanasia easier and promoting "death with dignity":* The B.C. Royal Commission on Health Care and Costs recommended amendments to the Criminal Code allowing a "competent adult patient" to refuse medical treatment and allowing a physician to prescribe "therapeutically necessary pain relief medication" that may be fatal;
- *Rationing by age:* Ontario ministry officials have released trial balloons about formally (as opposed to informally, now) refusing bypass surgery and other high-cost treatments to those over a certain age. After all, they restrict many procedures to the elderly in other quite civilized countries!
- *Cutting down on currently available benefits:* Cutting drugs from the Ontario Drug Benefit Plan;
- *Closing acute-care beds and "using the money saved for long-term-care facilities, home care, and free-standing clinics":* Sounds logical, the bed cuts have been made in province after province, but don't hold your breath waiting for those new facilities and new services – they cost money. The burden of care is effectively being shifted to the private sector (you and me) while the Good Ship Universal Medicare sails serenely on.

It used to be that a clear majority of the poor were older women. Increasingly the poor are children, especially the children of single-parent families. Today's elderly grew up during the Great Depression and are used to doing without. Tomorrow's elderly have never really known anything but our Medicare and are the most aggressive and fussy consumers the world has ever known. Everyone gives lip service to the contributions of the elderly in building our prosperity. How are we as a society going to balance their needs with the needs of new generations?

Limited Ability to Pay: What Will Medicare Continue to Cover?

The subject of this discussion can no longer be: "Everything should be covered." Oddly, many Canadians seem to persist in deluding themselves that "All of It" can be covered (when it isn't now and really never has been) and to demand that "The Right to Health" be carved in constitutional stone. Canada's health system is wounded. To use a medical analogy, the patient is exsanguinating (bleeding-out) and there is little time for debate. Decisions must be made on the fly. The Medicare experiment was great while it lasted, but it is not capable of continuing in the same form. We are collectively out of money. Something has to go! Whomever you believe in the endless arguments about "waste," "we have enough money if managed properly," "let's find private sources of funding," "user fees," we are still faced at the moment with closing beds, closing some hospitals, caps on doctors' incomes, maldistribution of doctors, and fewer medical services totally covered by the one third-party payer, the government.

Even if we are able to decrease wastage, we will not eliminate it. Do you ever throw out food at home that has gone bad no matter how carefully you shop and plan your household meals? In Canada's agricultural system, for example, about 25% of everything produced eventually is wasted. Is every visit to a shaman necessary or effective? The best managed system in the world is not going to materialize overnight, and ideal efficiencies and cost-effectiveness do not happen without a cost. Few of the needed system management tools are yet in place.

Referendum, national or provincial? Cuts mandated arbitrarily by health policy experts and medical professionals? National consensus in Canada, even if achievable, will take longer than we have time for. Someone, likely health ministry officials, is already making arbitrary decisions. Regionally, there are examples of reversals from previously entrenched positions. In Ontario, the health ministry has recently been reviewing a number of programs, and one particularly, the Ontario Drug Benefit Program (ODBP) for senior citizens. Arbitrarily, as decided by internal ministry review, and in significant numbers, drugs previously covered are being delisted. It is expected that the current list of some 2,500 drugs will be reduced to less than 500 at the end of this review process.

If items can be removed from a drug formulary this easily, where's the problem in setting up a similar review panel to delist (selectively deinsure) medical services previously covered by Medicare benefits? This may be the easiest method of limited healthcare services' privatisation. The cost is simply shifted from a Medicare benefit to a personal expense, available from the private sector.

The citizens of the State of Oregon in the western USA have come up with a "list of what should be covered by their core health plan." We will examine it in more detail in the next chapter. It is not as all-encompassing as the Canadian package. Forced to make some tough choices, they have been able to prioritize a list, however imperfect. This book is partly about making choices. It will continually be emphasized and reemphasized throughout this book, that the author firmly believes modern medical science has outstripped any society's ability to create a single global method of payment for all these things. Every day the engine of technological change is broadening this gap.

CHAPTER 3

SHOULD CANADA CONSIDER GOING DOWN THE OREGON TRAIL?

The Oregon Experiment: A Precedent For Others to Follow?

We have begun to recognize in Canada that all publicly funded health programs suffer a common problem: the range of human ingenuity applied to healthcare now exceeds the known capacity to pay for it. The effects of this disparity are bound to be unpleasant. Not everyone will receive the healthcare from which they might benefit; there will be suffering and death that could have been avoided or postponed. Choices must be made. The hard word is rationing. The problems of healthcare rationing occupy, and will continue to occupy, an increasing amount of space in professional as well as lay media.

The State of Oregon has wrestled with all of this in attempting to find a direction, and the resulting process has intriguingly and deservedly drawn world attention. [1] This attention is not for simply biting the bullet and making hard choices about how much care they can afford to provide their citizens. Unwittingly, and perhaps without being aware of it, Oregon is the first government and population to start to come to terms with realities forced by the healthcare paradigm shift. Recognizing that government can never pay for all available health interventions, they have begun the differentiation of the entire domain of "healthcare interventions" into different segments, essential and less essential. They may not know it yet, but their's is only the first attempt of limited economies to try and contend with the future: To come to terms with the new order of the health market, which will grow indefinitely in size and scope.[2]

The system in Oregon is very different from ours. The state population of 2.7 million has some 450,000 citizens (17%) with absolutely no healthcare insurance. The rest of Oregonians (the majority – 83%) are covered to some extent by private plans which may or may not be employer-funded or by Medicaid and Medicare programs for welfare recipients and senior citizens. Like health coverage in many parts of the United States, it is a patchwork quilt of care. The 17%, or "deserving working poor," are the target of the new insured coverage proposals – often referred to as the "Oregon Experiment." The Oregon process (to be described below) has generated one of the more innovative approaches to this worldwide problem seen in the past three decades, as well as explosive debate.

As Oregon moves (this is not yet a *fait accompli*) towards a somewhat contracted version of what we now have in Canada, in which "the working poor" are covered by health care that is partly publicly financed, the question of what types of services will be insured became in-es-capable. Canadians are just now barely beginning to realize that government funding of it all is impossible. The Oregon approach has been to devise a list (709 services and treatments) of healthcare priorities based on three principles: equity for those now not insured; explicit choice (fairer than hidden rationing); and a combination of expert analysis and community values. One strategy – the scientific – is to rank services according to qualities of well-being and cost-benefit. Another, more innovative, is to go to the public for ideas through community meetings and a telephone survey, a procedure made mandatory by state legislation. The public ranked quality of life, prevention, ability to function, cost-effectiveness and equity in this order.

The Process: 47 Community Meetings

In 1989 an eleven-member commission comprised of physicians and consumers was established. Their job was to develop a prioritized list based on the effectiveness of the services. Since there is no perfect data on outcomes yet, they brought together panels of physicians to consider what their experience has taught them about what works and what does not. They had forty-seven community meetings around the state for the public to talk about their opinions on what was important in making decisions about health resources allocations. They spent a total of 25,000 volunteer hours in developing the list. The list is comprised of what they describe as "'condition treatment pairs," as treatments for varying conditions have different effectiveness.

Under the Oregon Plan, health care services are divided into three types: (a) essential; (b) very important; and lastly, (c) "valuable to certain individuals" but significantly less likely than the first two to be cost-effective or to produce long term gain.

OREGON PLAN'S CATEGORIES OF CARE

Rank	Condition and effects of treatment	Examples
1	Acute fatal, prevents death, full recovery	Appendicectomy; treatment for myocarditis
2	Maternity care, including disorders of the newborn	Obstetric care of pregnancy; treatment for low birthweight babies
3	Acute fatal, prevents death, without full recovery	Treatment for bacterial meningitis; reduction of open fracture of joint
4	Preventive care for children	Immunisations; screening for vision or hearing problems
5	Chronic fatal, improves life span and patient's wellbeing	Treatment for diabetes mellitus and asthma; all transplantations
6	Reproductive services	Contraceptive management; vasectomy
7	Comfort care	Palliative treatment for conditions in which death is imminent
8	Preventive dental care	Cleaning and flouride
9	Proved effective preventive care for adults	Mammograms; blood pressure screening
10	Acute non-fatal, treatment causes return to previous health state	Treatment for vaginitis; restorative dental service for dental caries
11	Chronic non-fatal, one time treatment improves quality of life	Hip replacement; treatment for rheumatic fever
12	Acute non-fatal, treatment without return to previous health state	Relocation of dislocated elbow; repair of corneal laceration
13	Chronic non-fatal, repetitive treatment improves quality of life	Treatment for migraine and asthma
14	Acute non-fatal, treatment expedites recovery of self limiting conditions	Treatment for diaper rash and acute conjunctivitis
15	Infertility services	In vitro fertilisation, microsurgery for tubular disease
16	Less effective preventive care for adults	Dipstick urinalysis for haematuria in adults under age 60; sigmoidoscopy for people under age 40
17	Fatal or non-fatal, treatment causes minimal or no improvement in quality of life	Treatment for end stage HIV disease; life support for extremely low birthweight babies (<500 g)

Figure 3

Essential services, categories 1 to 9, (Categories of Care, *Figure 3*) include those that preserve life, maternity care, preventive care for children and adults, most reproductive services and comfort care for terminally-ill patients. Very important services (categories 10 to 13) include treatment for non-fatal conditions for which full or partial recovery is expected or for which treatment will improve the quality of life.

Services that may be valuable to certain individuals (categories 14 to 17) include those for nonfatal conditions not responsive to treatment, heroic treatments for infertility, and for conditions in which the quality of life is little improved by treatment. Much more interesting than what is included under "essential" and "very important" is what is included under the third heading, "valuable to certain individuals," because such items are not funded by the plan (*Figure 4*).

HEALTHCARE VALUABLE TO CERTAIN INDIVIDUALS

Examples of some conditions for which health care services are deemed "valuable to certain individuals" and may not be paid for under the Oregon Plan follow:

Category	Examples
Conditions that get better on their own	Viral hepatitis, common cold, viral sore throat, minor head injury (bump on the head)
Conditions for which a "home" treatment is effective (eg: applying an ointment, not using a painful leg, applying hot packs and drinking plenty of fluids	Sprain, hives, canker sore, non fungal diaper rash, food poisoning
Conditions for which treatment is not generally effective, is futile or is essentially "heroic"	Surgery for low back pain, severe brain injury, aggressive medical treatment for the final stages of cancer or acquired immune deficiency syndrome (AIDS) (comfort care such as pain management and hospice care is provided for these patients) or for extremely premature babies

Figure 4

The Oregon Plan assumes everyone is entitled to a diagnosis as part of the standard benefits package. Once the diagnosis is established, coverage for treatment is determined by the position of the condition on the list of 709 ranked condition-treatment pairs.

All of this resulted in blending groups of illnesses, conditions and procedures, into a final detailed list. The level of funding determined by the state legislature will determine the cut-off point in the list; conditions and procedures above the line will be insured and those below will not. The cut-off point could move up or down over time, depending on the availability of funds. As of this writing the cut-off point was somewhere around 587 in the list. As a matter of interest, line 587 includes the last item, covered "Esophagitis." The entire process is under the control of an appointed commission that is independent of politics.

Critics have made much of the fact that this plan might result in the payer (taxpayer) setting limits for the deserving poor with an excess of cautious paternalism. One of the most publicized decisions was not to fund organ transplantation (although kidney transplantation is covered by Medicaid at present). It is worth noting that Britain's National Health Service does not pay for transplants above age 50, or for renal dialysis above 50. Whether the entire proposal will come to pass depends on negotiations between state and federal governments over the financial details. At this moment, all the appropriate Oregon Bills necessary to make the Plan law have been passed. $35 million has been set aside by Oregon. Before the plan can go into effect it needs federal government approval to change Oregon State Medicaid guidelines, because some people currently receiving Medicaid must lose some benefits.

Decisions on healthcare rationing are made in Canada all the time but not by explicit public choice. Some are made by politicians (where a hospital is located, how it is equipped). Some are set out by legislation, as in the province-wide introduction of non-ionic radiographic contrast media (an injectable substance used in kidney X-rays to enhance pictures of the urinary collecting system) in Ontario. Some are made more diffusely as doctors move away from forms of medical practice (e.g. anaesthesia and rural obstetrics) perceived as bearing too high a risk for a negligence lawsuit.

Nowhere in Canada do we have a system that continually samples public opinion and community values about priorities in healthcare. If we want to carry out the provisions of the Canada Health Act in the future, we will have to make explicit decisions concerning costs and benefits within a publicly presented, standard benefits plan.

A decision from Washington is still pending as to whether the Oregon proposal will be given legislative and economic approval. There is much contention about this plan, as a precedent to many other cash-strapped state economies is very much anticipated. Approval for Oregon may be the signal for a wave of health reforms. Defenders of the plan remind critics that this list simply articulates what is actually happening right now in practice! They also remind everyone that the plan is not a substitute for National Health Care Reform. Only a temporizing move. Currently, the rumour around Washington, D.C. is that the Bush Administration will in fact kill the proposed Oregon Plan. It is believed that passage would be perceived as "insensitive" in an election year. As we went to press, it was learned that in mid-August, 1992, the Bush administration did indeed reject the Oregon Plan, sending it back for an overhaul. This overhauling process will delay the issue until after the presidential election in November.

The lesson for Canada from the Oregon Experiment is that the medical profession and the public may have to use a similar process to decide what we will cover in our Medicare plan, and what will not be covered. Additionally, we must develop some kind of fast track method of determining what is appropriate from what is inappropriate healthcare. We must develop a "real time" outcomes methodology, as things are moving too fast for long range determinations.

Diagnosis Shift, Specialty Shift

If we ever get to the situation where Canadians opt for an Oregon Plan list of government insured and non-insured services, there may be longer term ramifications which are still hard to predict. The flaw in the Oregon Plan as it currently exists is that everyone is entitled to a diagnosis. This may result in doctors making a diagnosis shift in marginal conditions so that an "Oregon-acceptable diagnosis" is always made if there is any doubt. Nevertheless this model is a useful reference point for making rational choices as to what might be covered and what not.

Those services not covered will have a decided effect on the ultimate supply of doctors that decide to go into the specialties not covered. We will not know until the future and such a list arrives! People's health seeking habits may remain the same, decrease, or increase in seeking care from the uncovered doctors. If demand for a specialty decreases, in the long run, medical students will not pursue those careers. The lag time is delayed of course. Currently dermatology pays well. If it did not, fewer would enter this field. All of these outcomes can be by design, of course.

Is Rationing Inevitable in Canada?

The short answer to this question is yes. Evidence from all health systems suggests that rationing takes place either covertly or explicitly and always has. Comprehensive healthcare, as hoped for by Lord Beveridge, free at the point of delivery, funded out of taxation and self-leveling, was an unattainable dream.

Every single health system management method as yet devised has been tried and has failed, or is failing for all the reasons this book discusses. All forecasts of health care expenditure show an ever expanding demand and exponentially increasing cost function.

There may be some hopeful signs recently. Improvements in surgical techniques are bringing down costs as flexible optical "scopes" become a trend in decreasing the impact of surgery on hospital bed usage and patient time-to-recovery. Just a few examples include the increasing

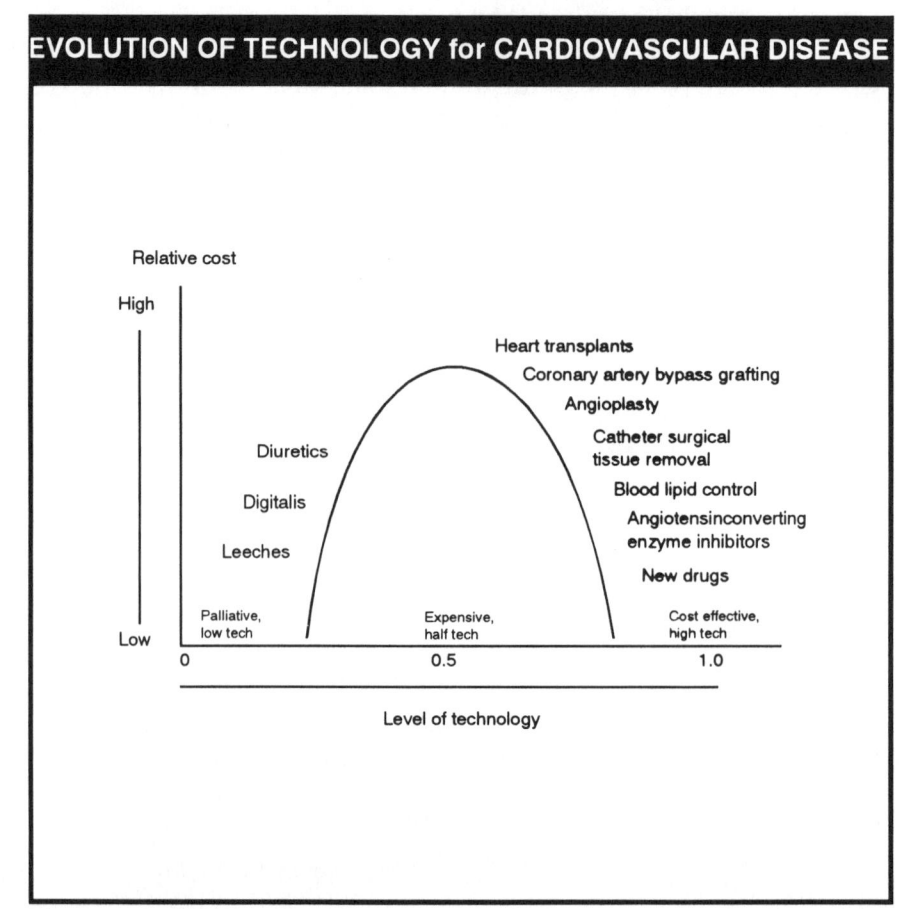

EVOLUTION OF TECHNOLOGY for CARDIOVASCULAR DISEASE

Relative cost

High

- Heart transplants
- Coronary artery bypass grafting
- Angioplasty
- Catheter surgical tissue removal
- Diuretics
- Blood lipid control
- Digitalis
- Angiotensinconverting enzyme inhibitors
- Leeches
- New drugs

| Palliative, low tech | Expensive, half tech | Cost effective, high tech |

Low

0   0.5   1.0

Level of technology

Figure 5

use of arthroscopic surgery of the knee and other joints; laparoscopic gynecological surgery via navel and other tiny abdominal incisions; and the replacement of gallbladder surgery by laparoscopic methods. We can expect a landslide of new "remote manipulation" optically-assisted techniques to develop. *(Figure 5)*.

Also, pharmaceutical developments are reducing or eliminating the need for surgery. A recent example is the current clinical trials underway which indicate that one or several drugs may eliminate surgery in men for benign prostatic hypertrophy (noncancerous prostate gland enlargement), one of the most common male problems currently requiring surgery.

Even Professor Jane Fulton, a health economist at the University of Ottawa and a frequently-quoted champion of our current system, stated on a CBC television interview, April 18, 1992, that rationing in Canada along the lines of the Oregon proposals is likely.

More and more people are discovering the importance of the lesson of Oregon for all governments. Simply, it is the democratic deciding of what is essential healthcare, less essential care and relatively unessential care and what we can afford to pay for. This is what all governments are going to have to do before long.

CHAPTER 4

WHAT SHOULD MEDICARE DO FOR PATIENTS?

Insurance Against CATASTROPHIC Illness

All national health insurance programs sprang from the altruistic and eminently humane principle of preventing accidental or catastrophic illness from bankrupting an individual and his/her family. Also understood at the time, and integral to such programs, was that the well greatly outnumber the ill, and thus it could be demonstrated by actuarial mathematics that the majority (the well) could subsidize the minority (the unwell). This reasoning was at the foundation of all national schemes.

It was never intended or anticipated that, driven by the impact of The Information Age and many other forces, catastrophic healthcare would come to include all forms of ill-health, from simple colds and stubbed toes to all forms of mental ill-health, notes from the doctor to excuse absence from work, joint replacement operations, the saving of most spinal cord injured patients, the saving of very tiny premature babies, and finally, the provision of coronary by-passes for every patient with heart artery narrowing (50% of North Americans).

The architects of Canadian Medicare were politicians, not actuaries. Thirty years ago the advances medical treatment would make in the intervening years were inconceivable. The impact of the current paradigm shift was not even imaginable. In the context of the present very broad definition of healthcare coverage, and in spite of reason telling us a single form of Medicare can't conceivably pay for it all, not just the FEW, but EVERY individual wants and is entitled to a piece of the healthcare pie, as long as EVERYBODY is paying for it.

This state of affairs is inconsistent with the laws of actuarial science. Also, part of the grand conception was that there be no discrimination against old people, those in dangerous occupations, the congenitally sick, the genetically impaired, those in other insurance schemes classified as the uninsurable. In this formulation there was no concept of individual risk or penalizing predisposition to illness. Thus, individual premiums (no longer present in most provincial plans) for Medicare were not weighted, and do not take into account those factors which predispose certain persons to a higher likelihood of having certain health problems than others by virtue of age, occupation, smoking, life-style etc. So the foundation on which every other insurance scheme is based was replaced by one with unlimited access and no adjustment in individual health coverage premiums. It is no wonder there is no personal incentive for wellness, prevention, or rational use of the system.

To complicate the situation further, as more and more types of non-catastrophic illness, or even worried wellness, gradually became reasons for seeking medical attention, no one (patient, healthcare provider, or politician) was prepared to take their political life in their hands and stand up and declare: "Hey, many of these people are not even sick let alone catastrophically ill!"

Even worse, non-physician healthcare providers of every stripe (chiropractors, reflexologists, naturopaths, herbalists, physiotherapists, massage therapists, psychologists, podiatrists, midwives, etc.) started to line up to get in on the action. After all, it's unfair for medical doctors to have the only claim on the health funding trough! So much for any rational attempt to try and come up with baseline coverage definitions of what might be called essential healthcare services.

The above paragraph might appear light-hearted, and in truth some of this has become laughable, but as time goes on and entrenched interests take hold, it is more and more difficult if not impossible to come up with definitions of what constitutes catastrophic or essential care, or even effective health services. That is why Ivan Illich, seeing so clearly in 1976 that things would turn out so badly, tried to raise the red flag of warning in his book, *Limits to Medicine*. He predicted that the doctors would redefine everything to be an illness! But it was hardly fair to blame everything on the much-maligned medical profession; WE ALL had a part in it.

Thus, universality, the philosophy that everyone has access to care, no one suffers, was naively thought possible, given the bogus actuarial theory that the well could subsidize the ill and the belief that, like the socialist state, illness would gradually waste away. There was no scientific way to prove or demonstrate this at the inception of Medicare, and now everyone passionately believes in it, regardless of the national deficit or a consensus to pay more taxes. **We in Canada have become far more concerned with our entitlement to healthcare than to whether we can actually afford such services.** The result is an all-but-infinite demand for healthcare. (Insurers and economists call this phenomenon moral hazard.) A very successful marketing job has been done on the concept of universal healthcare coverage. We have given the public and the profession the keys to the nation's candy store. Hardly anyone even wants to chase them out!

It's No Fun to Say No

No Canadian politician dared to tamper with the healthcare system in any way until about 1985 when the federal Conservatives decided to say enough is enough. In a nut shell, they decided that 9% of the GNP was more than enough funds to contribute to the national health plan. Also, the federal government stated that it was the provinces' responsibility to deal with structural problems, funding problems, and the problem of regional demand and its local cost. And so they initiated changes in the federal transfer of funds that culminated in spring 1991 with Bill C-69 which froze funding at 1989-1990 levels. They also determined to hold the line until at least 1995. Bill C-69 did not say they would indefinitely continue the freeze, or that they would reduce previous funding levels.

The chorus of howls (spelled HEAL – Health Action Lobby) that has risen, from the provinces and HEAL, about the imminent end to Medicare, has continued since then. HEAL wants Medicare entrenched in constitutional law as a right. Included in the HEAL group are: The Consumers' Association of Canada (CAC); The Canadian Hospital Association (CHA); The Canadian Long Term Care Association (CLS); The Canadian Medical Association (CMA); The Canadian Nurses' Association (CNA); The Canadian Public Health Association (CPHA); and The Canadian Psychological Association (CPA). Some critics believe the federal moves were too precipitous, passed on the sly, when public attention was riveted on the Gulf War, etc. Clearly, it is not fun to say no.

It is appropriate at this point to examine why the federal government might have decided that 9% of the GNP is a reasonable or affordable amount of the nation's wealth to spend on healthcare. Most analysts believe that no additional health benefits seem to accrue (using standard indicators of national well-being: infant mortality; life expectancy at birth, etc.) to nations when they spend in excess of 10%. In fact, the

United States is now spending almost 13% of its GNP on health (and rising) and although many Americans have arguably the best healthcare on earth, and clearly many of the most innovative health scientists and physicians of any system, 35 million have no health coverage, and polls of the American people indicate 85% support for a national healthcare system. (*Figure 6*)

Every country's government is now scrambling to reform their healthcare systems. Suddenly, governments want doctors to save money by becoming more innovative and imaginative. Suggestions range from shrinking numbers of services, entreating healthcare providers to properly perform the role of gatekeeper to the healthcare treasure chest, home and community care, cuts in the number of licensed practitioners and capping physician incomes, to placing all doctors on salary. These measures indirectly have the effect of rationing care, or denying care to some people. The buck gets passed from the federal politician, saying no to funding the health system, to the doctor saying no on the front lines. Few politicians dare tell patients to be fiscally responsible.

OECD HEALTH INDICATORS, 1989

	Life expectancy at birth (years)		Infant mortality (per 1,000 live births)	Health spending as % of GDP	Doctors per 10,000 population
	Male	Female			
Japan	75.9	81.8	4.6	6.7	16
Germany	71.8*	78.4*	7.5	8.2	30
United States	71.5	78.5	9.7	11.8	23
Britain	72.4*	78.1*	8.4	5.8	14
France	72.4	80.6	7.5	8.7	30
Canda	73.0*	79.8*	7.2*	8.7	22
Holland	73.7	80.0	6.8	8.3	24

*1988 and 1986 Source: OECD

Figure 6

Even doctors live in today's competitive world. Particularly in big cities where most of the doctors practice (too many according to most analysts), try telling a sick or not-so-sick patient what he/she does not want to hear: "No." This patient has expectations raised by our general sense of healthcare entitlement and also perhaps some specific health news item that caught his attention sufficiently to bring him to the doctor's office. Example: A government news promotion article recommends flu shots for people over 65 but the patient has misunderstood, is only forty, and does not fit the government guidelines for the shot. He's busy and doesn't want to take time out for flu. That's understandable. Facing "No," some patients will react by voting with their feet and finding a doctor who will deliver what they want. Thus, don't expect to find too many doctors acting prudently, and saying no. This scenario is less a problem in smaller communities, where many fewer doctors practice, and where the sheer numbers of patients flocking to them act as a disincentive to the more frivolous requests (demands) city doctors so frequently encounter.

Not all citizens make frivolous use of the system, but as the system is currently configured, it is just so easy to do. Before Medicare, there were few visits to doctors for notes, bruised knees, headaches, vague aches and pains, minor rashes, colds and flus, sniffles, fatigue, exercise advice, diet advice, living advice, etc. Yes, some doctors do pander and encourage every patient concern, inviting overutilization. Playing along is the path of least resistance, and it is good for business.

What Can Modern Medicine Do for Patients?

This topic could easily fill many books. Libraries and book stores are overflowing, not only with medical textbooks but with popular medical books on every illness and symptom known. It would be easier to make a list of what medicine cannot do.

There has been intensive effort by researchers and health analysts over the years to determine which, amongst the thousands of medical and surgical interventions currently available, are truly effective or efficacious. This so-called "outcomes" task has barely begun despite the pressure as health costs sky-rocket. It is a huge undertaking, and is very costly; it will take years to review existing services, let alone emerging technologies and techniques. No one can deny that it is essential that we eliminate what doesn't work, and retain that which does.

The placebo effect was mentioned earlier in the book. Doctors and patients all know that the placebo effect works. Should it be considered part of modern effective care or must it be expunged from the doctor's bag of tricks in the interests of cost containment? Currently less than five percent of all the things doctors do have been subject to the scientific scrutiny of a randomized clinical trial (RCT). The RCT is modern medicine's best statistical methodology for separating out the placebo effect from true inherent effectiveness. By this technique we attempt to filter out either the patient's (or the doctor's) preconceived notions or beliefs in the value of a specific therapy or medical intervention, from the actual efficacy of the intervention itself. A difficult task. In a randomized clinical trial (usually of a new drug, but increasingly of procedures), neither the doctor nor the patient know whether they are receiving the true drug or the dummy or placebo. Here, "placebo" is used as a term for a pill that looks like the real thing, but contains only sugar or other non-active agent. In this way the RCT process neutralizes any expectation that the agent under trial has healing power.

The NIH Consensus Development Program

In the U.S. in 1977, the National Institute of Health's (NIH) Consensus Development Program made a start on the task of separating effective practices from useless ones, by examining, initially, the most common medical services and proposing "consensus guidelines" for their optimal management. These common services are not necessarily high technology, and most items were chosen because they are used so frequently at some point in our lives. Please note that consensus guidelines are not necessarily identical to guidelines distilled from RCTs. Also note, consensus guidelines do not necessarily address the issue of whether or not the procedure or treatment under study is truly effective. However, consensus guidelines represent about as good a standard of care as medical science is able to develop at this time. The table below *(Figure 7)* is a listing of conferences and subjects examined to date.[1]

One can see that even this relatively short list of common problems far from exhausts the number of possible medical interventions that might be made the focus of a consensus-forming process, let alone things that medicine can do for patients. Another chronic problem with consensus-forming guidelines is that once the consensus guideline is drafted, it is out of date unless constantly updated. More confusing, there are a rapidly proliferating number of guidelines appearing and doctors are reacting with confusion and increasing scepticism about which to follow.

The diffusion of these types of guidelines into regular medical practice is increasingly becoming the responsibility of Quality Assurance administrators in hospitals.

Canada tends to utilize other countries' consensus experience research, as the cost of repeating such a process is prohibitive. Occasionally, where there is controversy or disagreement, Canada will assemble its own local panel of experts to draft a Canadian guideline. As an example, Canada did not agree with American cholesterol-screening guidelines and we developed our own (more conservative).

The only ideal, but not yet routinely available, method of maintaining the timeliness of such guidelines is to design an intelligent computer system that could continually "digest" a preselected set of literature titles as designated by the monitor group, and create an ongoing status

NIH CONSENSUS DEVELOPMENT PROGRAM

TOPIC	DATE
Breast Cancer Screening:	September, 1977
Educational Needs of Physicians and Public Regarding Asbestos Exposure:	May, 1978
Dental Implants: Benefit and Risk:	June, 1978
Mass Screening for Colorectal Cancer:	June, 1978
Treatable Brain Diseases in the Elderly:	July, 1978
Indications for Tonsillectomy and Adenoidectomy: Phase I:	July, 1978
Availability of Insect Sting Kits to Non-Physicians:	September, 1978
Mass Screening for Lung Cancer:	September, 1978
Supportive Therapy in Burn Care:	November, 1978
Surgical Treatment of Morbid Obesity:	December, 1978
Pain, Discomfort, and Humanitarian Care:	February, 1979
Antenatal Diagnosis:	March, 1979
Transfusion Therapy in Pregnant. Sickle Cell Disease Patients:	April, 1979
Improving Clinical and Consumer Use of Blood Pressure Measuring Devices:	April, 1979

Figure 7

NIH CONSENSUS DEVELOPMENT PROGRAM

TOPIC	DATE
The Treatment of Primary Breast Cancer; Management of Local Disease:	June, 1979
Steroid Receptors in Breast Cancer:	June, 1979
Intraocular Lens Implantation:	September, 1979
Estrogen Use in Postmenopausal Women:	September, 1979
Amantadine; Does it Have a Role in the Prevention and Treatment of influenza?	October, 1979
The Use of Microprocessor-Based Intelligent Machines in Patient Care:	October, 1979
Removal of Third Molars:	November, 1979
Thrombolytic Therapy in Thrombosis:	April, 1980
Febrile Seizures:	May, 1980
Adjuvant Chemotherapy of Breast Cancer:	July, 1980
Cervical Cancer Screening; The Pap Smear:	July, 1980
Endoscopy in Upper GI Bleeding:	August, 1980
Caesarian Childbirth:	September, 1980
CEA as a Cancer Marker:	September, 1980
Coronary Artery Bypass Surgery; Scientific and Clinical Aspects:	December, 1980
The Diagnosis and Treatment of Reyes Syndrome:	March, 1981
Computed Tomographic Brain Scanning:	November, 1981
Diet and Childhood Hyperactivity:	January, 1982
Total Hip Joint Replacement:	March, 1982
Clinical Applications of Biomaterials:	November, 1982
Critical Care Medicine:	March, 1983
Liver Transplantation:	June, 1983
Treatment of HyperTriglyceridemia:	September, 1983
Precursors to Malignant Melanoma:	October, 1983
Drugs and Insomnia:	November, 1983
Dental Sealants in the Prevention of Tooth Decay:	December, 1983

Figure 7

NIH CONSENSUS DEVELOPMENT PROGRAM

TOPIC	DATE
Diagnostic Ultrasound in Pregnancy:	February, 1984
Abalgesic-Associated Kidney Disease:	February, 1984
Osteoporosis; Treatment and Prevention:	April, 1984
Mood Disorders; Pharmacologic Prevention of Recurrences:	April, 1984
Fresh Frozen Plasma; Indications and Risks:	September, 1984
Limb Sparing Treatment of Adult Soft Tissue Sarcomas and Osteosarcomas:	December, 1984
Lowering Blood cholesterol to Prevent Heart Disease:	December, 1984
Travelers Diarrhea:	January, 1985
Health Implications of Obesity:	February, 1985
Anaesthesia and Sedation in the Dentists Office:	April, 1985
Electroconvulsive Therapy:	June, 1985
Adjuvant Chemotherapy for Breast Cancer:	September, 1985
Smokeless Tobacco Use; Health Implications:	January, 1985
Prevention of Venous Thrombosis and Pulmonary Embolism:	March, 1986
Integrated Approach to Pain Management:	May, 1986
Plasmaphoresis in the Treatment of Neurological Diseases	June, 1986

IN PROGRESS

Visual Impairment Due to Cataracts in the Aging Eye

Diagnosis and Treatment of Benign Prostatic Hypertrophy

Treatment of Prostate Cancer

Pain Management

Optimal Management of Acute Myocardial Infarction

Optimal Management of Chronic Coronary Artery Disease

Diagnosis and Treatment of Depressed Outpatients in Primary Care Settings

Delivery of Comprehensive Care in Sickle Cell Disease

Prediction, Prevention, and Early Treatment of Pressure Sores in Adults

Urinary Incontinence in the Adult

Figure 7

report. This is under investigation in other disciplines (physics, chemistry, biology) and must still be considered esoteric artificial intelligence (AI) research. Researchers are working on computer software (electronic surrogates or agents) that will act like a librarian, keeping track of certain types of scientific literature without human supervision. Such systems are not available yet for medicine.

In Canada, some of the provinces have just begun creating guidelines for medical care as part of Quality Assurance, as a means of keeping what works and eliminating that which is wasteful or of questionable value. We have a very long way to go in this important but costly and very time consuming and process. We must also keep in mind that the process of eliminating what doesn't work will never be completed!

A View from the Other Side:
A Previous Ontario Minister of Health Speaks Out

In a very interesting luncheon conversation recently, MPP Elinor Caplan, formerly Ontario's Minister of Health, strongly opposed my suggestion of a dual system (both Medicare and private sector healthcare in parallel) by insisting that the government can afford to deliver all the effective care the public needs within Medicare if patients only received health services that were effective, and we eliminated the rest. She continued to make the point that current figures of waste (25-30%) in the system were probably very conservative. Thus, she believes that allowing the public to access private sector health services (entrepreneurial medicine) for ineffective (or uninsured), or questionably effective services would be tantamount to encouraging people to waste money. We did not get into a discussion of where the placebo effect fits in her scheme of things. Nor did we discuss a range of medical services that are effective but, according to some, not essential.

The entire spectrum of cosmetic surgical interventions is a complex and contentious subject. Meme and silicone breast implants (the current controversy raging around this procedure, notwithstanding) and interventions like body-shaping liposuction are popular medical services. Cosmetic surgery is not part of Medicare, as it is considered non-essential, but few could describe the results of such services as ineffective.

As we have shown, if it were so easy to define what is effective, and not effective, we would not be in the mess we're in now! While we can all agree that patients should receive only effective care, our current ability to discriminate is very incomplete. The whole concept of "effective" as opposed to "ineffective" is seriously flawed. Health services are neither black or white. There are shades of gray.

The Hon. Elinor Caplan further made the point that medically knowledgeable or informed patients would better understand what was effective as opposed to ineffective and probably decide on the former. However, many doctors are currently delivering services they truly believe are effective which some researchers would deem ineffective. If the doctors who are supposedly informed don't know, how are the patients to know?

None of this is intended to deny or oppose recent new health perspectives by government that properly recognize that general public health and wellbeing involve much more than the availability of currently available healthcare services and doctors. There is no question that physical and social environments, genetic endowment, safe employment, living styles, and many other factors are also important. Some would say, however, that this view, that they can be improved, is a wonderful ideal, forever pursued, forever elusive, impractical, and impossible to implement nationally, due to human nature and more importantly, due to cost.

CHAPTER 5

WHAT SHOULD MODERN MEDICINE DO FOR PATIENTS?

Our Medical Moral Imperative

As little as ten years ago most severe spinal cord injuries resulted in the immediate or early death of the patient. Every year in North America, as many as 20,000 people receive injuries from accidents which result in spinal cord injuries paralyzing them from the neck down. In Canada, three patients every single day, usually as a result of a hockey injury or a dive into shallow water, or an automobile accident, end up in a wheelchair as a result of an irreversible spinal cord injury.

As recently as five years ago, those not dying outright from their injuries could expect to spend the rest of their lives wheelchair bound, with very limited prospects for any type of productive rehabilitation. Since 1986, aggressive acute care treatment of the spinal injury, together with the use of very costly high tech imaging, has allowed doctors to identify the exact level and degree of injury, and save the lives of most of these patients. In the past several years there has also been a revolution in the rehabilitation of such patients. While most of those with serious spinal injuries must still use wheel chairs, a growing number are beginning to contemplate some degree of reversal of their paralysis and reclaim previously irretrievably lost motor function. Intensive research is under way to discover how to regenerate spinal connections and, failing this, to teach patients to maximize their remaining healthy spinal cord to develop motor skills not possible just a few years ago.

These wonderful achievements bring hope to these disabled patients, and tremendous pride to the rehabilitation health professionals who have made such strides in care. So, 20,000 people who would previously have died now utilize a host of costly services unavailable a few years ago. If these people lived in a Third World country, they would still die today. The Moral Imperative of our society insists that if medical technology can save or improve life it must do it. And so we now must struggle with the fact that such measures are contributing to the possible bankruptcy of a system that never anticipated such developments. The lesson from this example is that unlike most other medical interventions that are only needed once (appendectomy, gallbladder removal, hysterectomy), the saving of a patient with neck-injury related paralysis WILL require MANY interventions as science makes possible improved mobility for these patients.

Correcting genetic defects and related illnesses has long been only a dream for medical intervention. That we might be able to prevent, let alone correct, such problems was until recently a distant Holy Grail. Such defects were God's will or "Man had no right to tamper with nature's decisions." Now, with a speed that is bewildering, biologists are developing a growing number of tests to detect some of these crippling and slowly lethal diseases in the foetus very early in pregnancy. The medical world (and the public) is now wrestling with the ethical problems this presents. Should a woman terminate a pregnancy known or likely to result in a child with, for example, Down's Syndrome, cystic fibrosis, spina bifida, muscular dystrophy (as this book was being completed, Canadian Medical Researchers in Ottawa isolated the gene causing myotonic muscular dystrophy), Tay-Sacs disease, etc.?

The world is facing a population time bomb. Not all genetic diseases (or "birth defects") result in early death, or traumatic physical or mental crippling, but many drag on, and at great cost to families and society. Is the government to decide in the interests of prevention, costs, and social engineering to "weed out" those unfortunates? This is scary stuff. Medicine will be able to detect such problems, long before it will be able to correct them or deal with the ethical problems.

What is clear from the forgoing material is that society clearly does not understand what we've put in motion with many of the successes of modern medicine. And we don't yet debate whether the system can afford a particular medical case before the ambulance arrives!

Currently, the Ontario government is grappling with how to pay for some of these types of treatments under their new "no fault" automobile insurance regulations.

The quandary for the future is to try and figure out whether all of this is a problem or an opportunity (my preference). Is the glass half empty or half full?

1. As a society we can't decide (and won't) not to provide new treatments. And yet, we have not considered the possible future imperative or "scenario of new treatment." Can we afford it, yes or no?
2. Should we not be looking at such interventions as an opportunity for the growth of new industries? For example, in effect, quadriplegia has become a new engineering industry.

Is the Hospital the Best Place to Deliver Healthcare? It Depends.

The answer to this question seems to change daily, and to depend on the rapid advance of medical science (or the depletion of the public purse). Hospitals are important and will continue to be so in spite of clear signals from provincial governments that the financial pressure they are putting on hospitals is here to stay, and that decentralization of care is a desirable long term goal.

Hospitals will continue to evolve and redefine themselves, as they have historically always done. Some will become very specialized, some general, some the hub of an expanding complex of services that probably will reach out to the home and other community care centres. Modern telecommunications and computers will accelerate these changes rapidly.

The modern hospital evolved out of a complex set of needs. Primarily it is/was an institution to deliver levels of care not available in offices, clinics, or homes. It is an institution where medical students and qualified doctors can continually educate and be educated in the latest methods. It is a place where 24-hour supervision by doctors and nurses can take place; a place where medically unstable patients can be stabilized before transfer to less intensive care; a place where procedures requiring individual specialists or teams of specialists not available under any other umbrella institution could be delivered. Finally, it is an institution where economies of scale justify and allow expensive, complex diagnostic and therapeutic tools to be made available: X-ray machines, CT-scanners, Magnetic Resonance Imagers, Diagnostic Ultrasound, and an endless variety of other expensive devices.

Healthcare experts also remind us that the current preeminent position of hospitals in our Canadian healthcare system arose in large part as a result of government funding, which has been, and to a lesser extent continues to be available to finance and encourage it.

As time went by, even general hospitals began to specialize and, with the exception of the smaller community or general hospitals, these larger urban general hospitals specialized into tertiary care hospitals. Such tertiary hospitals only perform complex high technology procedures like open-heart surgery, brain surgery, and joint replacement surgery. Tertiary hospitals tend to be found only in large cities, and usually are associated with a medical school.

Peter Drucker, an American management guru and writer, has called hospitals the most complex organizations yet created by humans. The cost of the staff required to support routine functions in modern hospital environments has resulted in unbelievable hospital daily rates ($1500-$2000 a day in many U.S. hospitals, typically $500+ per day in Canada). Administrators are now urgently attempting to decide which medical services can be shifted to less expensive facilities.

We have already seen that it is very difficult to choose, from an almost endless list of therapies and medical interventions, those that should be covered by some kind of health insurance or Medicare package. This author believes most citizens would like to be assured serious illness would always be covered. But even the definition of serious is subject to conflicting opinion. Perhaps those interventions requiring hospitalization are "serious." Unfortunately, even this arbitrary and broad guideline is fraught with complications as procedures previously only available in hospitals are being moved out to other types of facility: regular kidney dialysis for those in chronic kidney or renal failure; day surgery for intermediate level gynaecological surgery such as uterine endometrial ablation; laparoscopic gallbladder removal; chemotherapy for cancer; and patient administered intermittent pain relief are all being moved into clinics or the home.

Not all illnesses requiring hospitalization start with an obvious need for hospitalization. Some medical problems requiring hospitalization only come to light after one or more visits and tests at a doctor's office. Does this mean the office-based services should be subject to user-fees, co-payments or deductibles, and only hospitalization covered? This would result in people being admitted to hospitals for investigation, just to cover the bills.

It is all too well known, in Canada and elsewhere, that fee schedules and payment schemes ultimately dictate not only how a system will process patients but how patients are treated. In general, doctors in Canada hospitalize patients when they can no longer manage the case elsewhere. In the USA, with an oversupply of hospital beds and a predisposition to lawsuits for the most frivolous reasons, there is much broader and even unnecessary use of hospitals to manage patient problems. And, conversely, because private insurance or the patient, himself, is paying, many procedures only performed in hospitals in Canada are day-surgery in the U.S.

To make matters more confusing, in some regions, many expensive and sophisticated tests are available only in hospitals, whereas in other locales, such procedures are available in clinics. One can see why the health system in such a large and sparsely populated country as ours is so complex and subject to such a large variation in methodologies.

As well, as manufacturers constantly strive to make their health products smaller, less expensive, and easier to use by fewer personnel, many expensive diagnostic devices previously the domain of hospitals are migrating to free-standing specialty facilities outside the hospital. In the U.S. this has happened very quickly in imaging services. A few years ago, "imaging" meant only X-rays, but recently with the explosion in advanced imaging devices (CT-Scanners, Magnetic Resonance Imagers, Ultrasound Imagers) any one of these modalities or all might be available in an imaging facility. In fact, imaging procedures in the U.S., but not in Canada, are now available cheaper in specialized imaging centres, where waiting times are shorter than at hospital-based facilities. Increasingly, many services are cheaper to deliver outside hospitals, and cost is driving this migration.

The Canadian imaging approach is entirely different from the American. In the U.S., any entrepreneur willing to finance an imaging centre simply raises the funds and buys or leases an ultrasound device, a CT, or an MRI, or all. Then the facility is open for business. In Canada, provincial laws limit the licensing of expensive high-tech imaging facilities to specifically selected public hospitals only. That is precisely why there are delays or actual inability to obtain needed MRI services in most Canadian medical centres. That was the intention. In Ontario, for example, there is an Act controlling the licensing of MRI and CT. Even if one had the facility funded privately, the equipment available at the ready, the radiologists ready to interpret the imaging records, and the patients lined up to be imaged, without a license you are not allowed to bill the provincial plan, or bill clients or their insurance companies privately. This has effectively eliminated growth of any private sector imaging industry in Canada, and it is a national shame.

Faced with such a rapidly changing healthcare world, and subject to economic necessity, we can expect a growing number of health activities (e.g. abortions), until recently only the province of hospitals, to shift to community-based facilities. Not all of these services involve high technology. In fact home care, and "hospital in the home" care are decidedly low tech. Whether in the end, the overall cost of this shifting care delivery emphasis will be less than the current hospital-based system is anybody's guess. The heyday of the very large general hospital may be passing. Such institutions may be the health system equivalents of dinosaurs. In fact, hospitals are also, and not surprisingly, experiencing their own paradigm shift.

Government analysts believe that there is considerable local medical service duplication. Some are now recommending that up to 5% of small, "inefficient" community hospitals be closed and replaced with Community Health Centres. Ten percent of hospital beds would also be closed.[1] People with problems requiring higher levels of specialist care would be transported to regional hospitals where services are available. Thus a Newfoundland patient requiring an elective cataract operation might be transported to a Montreal hospital rather than treated locally. Naturally, this idea is not popular with the Newfoundland patient or his family. The closing of local hospitals or the downgrading of local hospitals to 12-hour clinics sparked demonstrations in New Brunswick. Even sending elderly patients fifty kilometres away is a serious hardship for them and their families and doesn't speak much to the need for "community."

However, if the public can accept this solution, and it can be proved that the overall cost of transporting patients to central facilities is much cheaper, this might be a solution to some of the problems of remote or smaller communities. However, many of these communities will say that this is what they have now, but that the current round of government cutbacks are making it much, much worse. In fact we are taking healthcare out of communities and thereby destroying those communities.

CHAPTER 6

MOTIVATING THE PARTICIPANTS

Motivating patients and care providers to be fiscally responsible is perhaps the most intractable challenge facing healthcare today. Solutions are not yet forthcoming. The patient or the public (until very recently) has never been the focus of cost-saving attention, and this is part of the reason we have come to our present circumstances. The focus has been on the health professional, primarily the physician, as the health cost ball starts rolling as soon as the patient-provider encounter takes place. In Canada it has been estimated that every practicing licensed physician, independent of their fees, on average, adds an annual cost component to the system of some $300,000-$500,000 in laboratory and associated tests. Even in Britain's National Health System (NHS), where almost every doctor is salaried, additional costs are incurred when a primary care physician (GP) refers a patient for laboratory tests, X-rays or other imaging procedures, or to a consultant or so-called secondary (general hospital) or tertiary (specialized hospital: cancer, cardiovascular surgery) care facility.

Doctors are increasingly being entreated to make prudent use of tests, as though we are collectively being imprudent. Medicine, to the great consternation and continuing disbelief of both the public and health administrators, still is, and will continue to be, a very unscientific art. The identical blood test on the same person on the same day in different labs may yield similar but considerably differing values. A German study reported in *Dtsch Med Wochenscheer* (115:408, 1990) noted that blood lipids (cholesterol) can vary considerably depending on whether the patient was lying or sitting when the sample was collected. Even the length of time the tourniquet is tightened on the arm can change blood values! Part of regular clinical judgment is to decide when and if ancillary tests are necessary, which ones, and how often. Is there waste? Absolutely. Might we collectively do better? Probably, given the knowledge and the desire. Much better? I doubt it.

The atmosphere within which healthcare providers work may be the most important factor in improving their attitudes towards cost-effectiveness. Relations between government and healthcare workers have deteriorated in recent years and as the economic crisis deepens, the rate of deterioration seems to accelerate. The endless cycle of blaming the participants has engendered tremendous ill feelings. It will take a lot of time and effort to repair the damage.

Why Should Doctors be Forced to Become the Gatekeepers?

By definition, the doctor is the patient's advocate or agent. His job is to do the best he can to diagnose, treat, and return the patient to normal functioning. If health resources are to shrink, the doctor's job will begin to include finding resources to do the treatment for the patients. Forcing the doctor into being both the forager as well as the gatekeeper of the healthcare treasure chest is a logical inconsistency as well as a conflict of interest.

If there was the necessary framework within which doctors could make both cost-effective and in-the-best-interests-of-the-patient decisions doctors would be more than happy to also be fiscally responsible. But such an ideal environment has not yet been created in Canada or the USA. In a speech reported in *Family Practice*, December 7, 1991, Robert Veatch, of the internationally renowned Kennedy Institute of Ethics (Washington, DC), recently told a mixed Toronto audience at a conference entitled "Tradeoffs in Health Care: The Ethical Implications," that he is alarmed by the move to conscript physicians into being gatekeepers of the health system.[1] He said, "I am convinced that we need a system that frees the clinician from any responsibility to be anything other than the patient's agent and simultaneously have a system of healthcare that will place limits on what is available to the clinician and will purposefully eliminate marginally beneficial services for the patients."

In Canada, doctors have heretofore been guided only by the moral imperative of the Hippocratic Oath, to do everything within their power to benefit the patient. No one has interfered in this. In the U.S., increasingly, an army of clerks and managers have been interposed between the doctor and his ability to carry out his obligations to his patient. Today in the U.S., even before the doctor begins to assess the patient, he/she must check what amount of insurance is available, and if costly tests or procedures are necessary, the doctor must first obtain clearance from risk managers. In a growing number of circumstances, such carte blanche clearance is denied and the doctor is not able to do what is necessary for the patient.

In an era where rationing is becoming a moral necessity, Veatch offers a twist to the Hippocratic Oath. Rather than empowering clinicians to benefit the patient according to his or her own ability and judgment, Veatch suggests a more objective standard of what constitutes a benefit be used. "We can no longer afford to rely only on the doctor's bedside intuition about what will benefit the patient. Individual clinical judgment is going to have to give way to collective (consensus) peer review of what the appropriate benefits are."

Clearly, the public must articulate the specific limits it wants placed on healthcare. The job of resource policing is going to have to fall to someone else, not healthcare providers. Working this out is what health ministry managers are paid to do. Novel and innovative incentive schemes will have to come from government, since they hold the monopoly. (In the Appendix there is an excellent recent editorial from the *Medical Post* on this subject.)

Cost-Effectiveness Tools in Health Delivery are Not Yet Available

Doctors and nurses are taught little about cost-effective strategies in patient management, as this has only recently been studied seriously in nursing and medical school curricula. The tools for assisting such practices are still emerging. An American hospital is in a much better position to assess cost-components of care in patient management than a Canadian hospital. The American system has operated for years with itemized billing for every single cost incurred by hospitalized patients. In an American hospital, typically, the staff counts every cotton swab, disposable syringe, plastic tube, cast material, and bandage used in the treatment of each patient. We have much to learn from this practice, and according to Dr. David Naylor, Assistant Professor, Faculty of Medicine, University of Toronto, we are ten years behind in this area.[2] Knowing what was spent is only the first step on the long road to knowing whether treatments are cost effective.

In any particular patient situation there are many possible paths to an appropriate diagnosis and treatment. Diagnosing and treating human beings continues to be a very unscientific process, for reasons beyond the control of medicine and government. Until healthcare system administrators can provide medical professionals with tools to manage patient care, entreating us to do the right thing is a relatively ineffective part of a yet very incomplete motivational strategy. Only recently, with the use of computers to track outcomes, has it been even remotely possible to come up with enough data to compare alternate diagnostic and therapeutic protocols and their respective success rates. It will be years before any Canadian province has the computer technology in place to provide the guidance needed by doctors to get optimal results cost-effectively.

We should be much further along in this type of systems implementation than we are. An article in *The Financial Post,* November 27, 1991, describes how difficult it was to get even a small Smartcard drug usage monitoring project up and running in the Windsor area recently.[3] A project involving 10,000 people which was to have started in February of 1991, was delayed until May because of software glitches associated with integrating Smartcard use with different local pharmacy computer systems. The main problem complicating the successful implementation of this Smartcard monitoring project was the lack of software standardization at different pharmacies. Each pharmacy had previously *(independently)* developed their own pharmacy software system. Thus, with the arrival of an external monitoring project, interfaces with different systems made progress that much slower.

Even if case management tools were provided, there must be an incentive system in place or no change will take place. A recent Rand Corporation study of the U.S. National Institute of Health's Consensus Development Program, on promoting change in medical practice habits, found that without very strong motivation to change existing physician habits, it just doesn't happen.[4] Education alone is not sufficient; there has to be a carrot or a stick!

In the matter of evaluating drug costs, for example, in Canada most physicians have no idea what a prescription costs unless the patient gives us feedback (rare). Before Medicare, patient and doctor made a joint decision about the most cost effective drug alternative based on the doctor's knowledge of price, efficacy and what the patient could afford. In those days there were many fewer drugs to keep track of, and they were much less expensive. With the widespread availability of generous drug plans funded by government or employee benefits packages, patients are even less concerned with prescription costs. It is not uncommon for patients to request doctors actually to add things to a prescription (vitamins, supplements) since they are covered by insurance. Witness the *Globe and Mail* editorial of December 3, 1991, "Suntan lotion and the cost of Medicare." Try and say no, and get a chilling look and occasionally lose the patient for attempting to be prudent! Only structural changes in the way patients pay dispensers for their medications appear to reduce costs. In Australia, for example, the first $15 of ALL prescriptions is the patient's responsibility to pay out of pocket with no reimbursement.

Another effective method of drug cost control has been to require the patient to pay for medications up front and get reimbursed by the plan later. This practical dollars out-of-pocket reality therapy alone has been proven in several provincial studies to make significant reductions (20%) in cost. All private drug benefit plans now require this approach. Other evidence shows that the introduction of users' fees or co-payment for drugs is effective in reducing costs. In spite of the fact that one province did a pilot study which revealed subsequent significant reductions in drug costs, this has not been widely followed. However, expect to see more of this one eventually.

Variable Patient Behaviour and Treatment Delays

Some patients by virtue of their personalities and experience practise exemplary preventive lifestyles and go to the doctor at the earliest sign of health problems. Others ignore symptoms, out of fear, denial or other personal reasons and delay seeking medical attention until it is very late in the progress of their disease. Such delays continue to happen in Canada though there is no no economic penalty for using health services. Such highly individual behaviours can, in some cases, create very different case outcomes (both in cost and success) for potentially the same problem, taking into account the considerably different genetic constitutions we each bring to a disease.

It is difficult to provide very specific examples of what can be delayed and what should not be, as we used not to be so obsessed with medical costs. It is going to take a long time to sort this out because similar diseases progress differently in different patients. For example, we can generalize that early detection and treatment of high blood pressure prevents stroke. We cannot, however, yet prove that it is cheaper. This is very complex. Prevention, as we will examine in more detail later, may cost much more than we currently realize. Again, for example, we can screen for breast cancer and pick it up much earlier. But, we do not, at present, have an adequate treatment plan for this condition. This frustrates doctors as much as patients, but that is the way it is at this time. The whole area of treatment options, and the role of watchful waiting, is just beginning to develop scientifically, and much needs to be done.

An interesting example highlighting the problem of delaying treatment was recently aired on an American Public Television program. The discussion ranged around the recent controversy about the Meme Breast Implant. Such surgically implanted devices have caused tremendous concerns among women for the long term deleterious effects, both of the external foam liner and of the potential release of small or large amounts of silicone contained within these prosthetic devices. These implants have been used for some time by healthy women seeking cosmetic breast size enhancement as well as for reconstruction in women who have had breast cancer surgery. What was alarming in this discussion was the comment by one woman advocate (in favour of such implants) that she had been told by many woman with established breast cancer that they would delay or avoid treatment for their breast cancer if cosmetic surgery (involving the implant of the Meme Device, or silicone implants) were not available to improve their appearance post-mamectomy (after cancerous breast-removal)!

Currently the entire issue of the Meme and Silicone Breast Prostheses has exploded in the media, and both the U.S. Food and Drug Administration (FDA), and Canada's Health Protection Branch has put the use of this product on hold pending FDA review. At the time this book left for the press, the expert committee in the USA advising the FDA were recommending an additional delay of sixty days before final decisions, and in the interim, that no silicone breast implants should be used for purely cosmetic applications (breast enlargement). Silicone implants can, however, still be used for the reconstruction of breasts removed as part of breast cancer operations. There has been no recommendation yet regarding the removal of existing silicone implants in healthy, symptom-free patients.

On April 16, 1992 Benoît Bouchard, the Minister of National Health and Welfare, Canada, announced his intention to maintain the moratorium for another six months on the distribution of silicone gel-filled breast implants.

Fiscal Responsibility for Patients

In spite of endless conflicting arguments by politicians, well-meaning socialists, and a host of academics, concerning the penalizing effects of any financial constraint to care-seeking (e.g. user fees), there is no absolute evidence which proves a patient cannot be economically motivated to make decisions to seek or not to seek medical attention in the same way they might chose any other commodity, product or service.

ENCOUNTERS AND ESTIMATED COSTS BY CONDITION OF PATIENT

	Number of Encounters	Per Cent of Encounters	Estimated Expenditures 1991-92
High Blood Pressure, Hypertension	903	5.6%	$87,004,874
Diabetes	361	2.2	34,467,332
Endocrine, Metabolic Disorders	142	0.9	16,579,522
Obesity	50	0.3	6,333,671
Arthritis, Bursitis, Tendinitis, etc.	1,359	8.4	134,528,406
Chronic Obstructive Lung Diesease, Chronic Bronchitis, Emphysema, etc.	274	1.7	26,606,231
Asthma	52	0.3	5,316,260
Prenatal Care	419	2.6	30,531,970
Heart Disease	751	4.7	76,113,846
Peripheral Vascular Disease	36	0.2	3,488,768
Anxiety, Stress	1,132	7.0	156,148,183
Headaches, Migraines	270	1.7	28,821,354
Upper GI Discomfort, Gastritis, Peptic Ulcer	547	3.4	57,111,957
Diarrhea, Lower GI Bleeds	259	1.6	27,277,653
Other Bowel Disorders	44	0.3	4,437,069
Conjunctivitis	92	0.6	7,941,147
Gynaecological Problems including Infection, Uterine Prolapse, etc.	1,055	6.5	118,924,741
Benign Breast Disease	37	0.2	4,351,337
Injury--Sports, MVA, Work	1,066	6.6	92,108,991
Infection--Genitourinary	333	2.1	32,098,329
Infection--Upper Respiratory	2,129	13.2	199,345,747
Infection--Ear	510	3.2	44,200,628
Infection--Other	816	5.1	72,471,985
Neurologic--CVA, Stroke, TIA	23	0.1	1,461,818
Neurologic--Hearing Loss, Vertigo	50	0..3	4,879,726
Neurologic--Epilepsy, Seizures	41	0.3	4,355,274
Neurologic--Other	65	0.4	6,664,728
Unspecified Allergy	191	1.2	10,312,337
Dermatological Problems	403	2.5	33,569,421
Anemia	57	0.4	4,363,585
Malignancy	70	0.4	7,334,461
Miscellaneous	319	2.0	33,413,179
Unspecified	2,269	14.1	227,434,092

Figure 8

This table first appeared in the January, 1992, issue of the *Ontario Medical Review* and is reprinted here with permission of the OMA.

In every aspect of daily life, citizens make choices based on economic constraints. Interestingly enough, they even live within these constraints when they spend hard-earned money up-front on alternative health professionals, as many alternative healers are not currently part of the health plan. People attempt to live within their means, and yet somehow they have been led by media and their political leaders (to a varying degree depending on party) to believe using the health system, in its broadest context, is different from shelter, food, education. This of course completely removes individual responsibility for healthcare, past, present, and future. The rationing is left to the providers. They have the distasteful task of trying to explain to patients and their families why some kind of action is not taking place.

Insurance companies set life insurance premiums depending on risk, based on an understanding of an individual's history, and no one thinks that non-smoker policies are unfair. But, wait, a minute, it's unfair to deny some people health insurance because they have bad genes! Everyone sympathizes with the intention of humane national health policies. These policies just happen to be bankrupting the nation.

Drink until your liver fails, then look for a transplant. Have a motor vehicle accident while intoxicated and maim or kill a few people, and then present yourself at the emergency room for treatment of your fractured hip – no accountability, no penalties of any kind for irresponsibility. Live a high risk lifestyle until a coronary bypass is needed. Eat until excess weight causes your hip and knee joints to crumble under the load; then, hey, where's the latest custom-designed titanium hip replacement? The list of self-induced illnesses is endless, but don't dare to punish the undeserving sick by creating some method of accountability. The problem of the undeserving poor and the undeserving sick will continue to confound moralists for a long time to come!

When Ontario Minister of Health, Frances Lankin, was asked by the panel moderator recently on TV Ontario's "Between the Lines" program whether or not smokers (a self-induced cause of illness) might not receive medical care as a result of government fiscal belt-tightening, she rapidly exclaimed, "Oh no, we would never consider doing something like that!" While absolute health service denial might not be the best measure in this particular example, one could reasonably inquire why some formula could not be devised that considered known health risk factors and penalized in some way those who practice unhealthy lifestyles. Or possibly reward those who practice healthy ones? Smokers are still 30% of the voting population!

In the U.S. the latest move by desperate corporate employers drowning in health benefit costs is to start dictating lifestyles to their employees. The NBC nightly news recently had a piece (September/91) on a growing number of employers who fire employees who smoke, drink alcohol, use drugs or weigh too much, as indexed statistics prove self-abuse (substance abusers, over-eaters, under-exercisers) incur higher sick-benefit payments! The immediate reaction, expected in litigious America, was for an obese ex-employee to sue his employer for infractions of human rights. A successful $450,000 settlement followed which clearly sets the stage for continuing lawyer employment. Beats working!

Of course, this couldn't occur in Canada, we're too humane, even though we can no longer afford our humane system. And whether or not we chose to believe it, our governments are looking more and more closely at some of the U.S. health management techniques (not so humane) to reduce costs in our system. Canadians call it managed care, resource allocation. Doctors call it rationing.

Flogging a Dread Public

"Practice preventive medicine or wellness measures." "Exercise more à la Participaction." "Stop smoking, don't drink." It is impossible to hide from the torrent of messages hurled at us about living a healthy lifestyle. Manufacturers of every kind of processed food have conceived clever ways of confusing you, the consumer, with the low content of whatever component is deemed bad for you.

Government subsidized communication programs have been increasingly successful in persuading us to get fit, eat correctly, stop abusing our lungs and livers, get appropriate check-ups and such. This is all excellent and should continue. But questions remain. Do such methods preach only to the converted, or about-to-be converted? How do we get to the hard core couch potatoes? No matter how many messages are broadcast to the public, a finite number will not answer the call. Do we in fact encourage more eating disorders (anorexia nervosa or bulimia) or other obsessive disorders with fitness and healthy lifestyle campaigns?

It is unlikely that the health promotion attempts of government can balance the infinite capacity of present day television and the popular press to stimulate our desire to get some of these technological and pharmaceutical health goodies. We examined the media's role earlier, in Chapter 2. Will public fear of global ecological changes drive ever greater use of the system? What do you think?

User Fees: Reality Therapy

User fees, while favoured by medical associations, are unpopular with politicians. Interestingly, they are not as unpopular with the public according to recent polls (70% in favour in one). Either side seems to be able to argue their case persuasively and to cite literature supporting the argument that such negative incentives work or don't work. An article in the *Toronto Star*, November 10, 1991 described an approach on user fees current in Sweden.[5] Canadians may be surprised to discover that even in Sweden people have to pay a small user fee for every health encounter: $9 for a primary care visit; $12 for a specialist visit; and $15 for an emergency department visit. Sweden is in the midst of an about-face in their health system experience, whereby the differential user fee is intended to drive patients to use the primary care sector rather than the secondary and tertiary levels for initial contacts. Similarly, Australia implemented a $2 user fee in January of 1991. The doctor must collect it from every patient for the government, and any missed collections are the doctor's expense!

Either we want universal access to healthcare or we don't. Proponents of user fees complain that patients come to emergency departments or doctor's offices for nothing more than handholding or reassurance. Is this not a legitimate function of medicine? Are user-fee advocates proposing that comfort or caring be excised from medical practice? Lacerations, fractures and ulcers are legitimate, but bereavement, anxiety and loneliness are not? On the same TV Ontario "Between the Lines" television program Professor Glen Beck, University of Saskatchewan, replied to Dr. William Goodman's (Toronto) point that, "Medicine is still 50% art and 50% science," by saying, "maybe we can't afford the art part." To which part of healthcare does the caring and comforting belong, in Professor Beck's view, the art part or the science part? Quebec has recently proposed the implementation of user fees to try and control abuse of hospital emergency departments, where most analysts agree only one in ten cases is a real emergency.

Creating a Market Economy within Medicine

In Britain, a 1989 revolutionary White Paper, "Working For People." has tried to create an internal healthcare system market economy in which certain types of services are purchased by Primary Care Physician Groups of certain sizes (general practitioners/GP). Thus the patient's

GP "buys" him the services of a surgeon at a hospital for his hip joint replacement. The GP shops around (far and wide apparently according to the plan) for an orthopaedic service that will deliver the aforementioned hip replacement at the best price, and with the least wait. Normal market forces are thus allowed to create competition amongst secondary care level suppliers (surgeons). It sounds great in theory, but has had implementation problems due to complexities of many kinds, including becoming an issue in the recent election.

In the early 1970s one unbelievable plan was proposed (possibly tongue-in-cheek) in a speech by the then Ontario Minister of Health to an audience of doctors at Toronto Western Hospital's weekly Grand Rounds. He said that in order to control the growing costs of medical tests (laboratory, X-rays, etc.), the doctors would have to pay for any test that did not turn out to be positive (which is usually less than 1 in 10)! A lot of doctors promptly walked out of the lecture! Let this Minister come to me if he suspects he has cancer! Perhaps he was going to establish a government fund to pay for liability suits.

The Patient as Gatekeeper?

Suggestions for encouraging personal fiscal responsibility have been floating around for a long while, but never seem to get implemented. One suggestion is to require the signature of the patient on every bill or chit submitted by the doctor to the provincial plan. The purpose of this process is two-fold: first, to stop doctors from charging for services not performed; and secondly, to make patients more aware of the cost of the encounter at point-of-service. This has been implemented in at least one region with minimal effect. Another suggestion is to send every citizen who has received any health service in the past three to six months an itemized statement listing all the costs paid by the Medicare plan on their behalf. Alberta currently does this, and continues to be as frustrated about costs as all the other provinces.

These devices sound reasonable on the surface, but let's examine them in more detail. First, the signature on the chit by the patient before submission. The idea is for the patient to authorize payment just as he does for any other transaction such as credit card purchases. This might have been useful in previous years, but since more and more billing is computerized, there eventually (soon) will be no paper bill to sign. Fifty-five percent of Ontario doctors currently send in a floppy disk with the month's patient-service invoices in magnetic form. Eventually transmission will happen on-line and even eliminate the disk. Also, who's going to pay the people who must look at and handle all those chits? If the purpose of getting patients to sign is to make them more aware of what they are costing the system, that is a useless exercise since the signing takes place after the service was delivered, and thus awareness of cost is after the fact and of little use motivationally.

As for the "periodic health services statement" as a mechanism for public motivation, once again, if the intention is to make patients and doctors more aware of cost, the timing of such motivational information should be before, not after, the service. Even if such an invoice was prepared by the doctor prior to service delivery, can you picture a patient looking at a list of what the doctor will do today, and associated costs, and deciding in the interests of fiscal prudence that the doctor leave out items 3, 5, and 7? Because patient payment is not immediate out-of-pocket, most analysts believe this method is futile. Finally, the government computer centres have more than enough to do just getting current patient bills paid, and a cheque sent to the physician. To add millions of additional reports to patients on their health bill audit trail would require equipment, mountains of paper and mailing costs. For so little motivational pay-off, it has not, and will not likely be implemented widely.

Incentives for Underservicing? No Way!

Every time one opens the newspapers lately one can find the same tired old conundrums about abuses of the health system by patients and doctors. The fee-for-service payment of doctors is increasingly under attack as one reason why there are incentives for over servicing the public. Strangely, there never seem to be any recommendations for methods of rewarding doctors for underservicing or declining to provide service. In a *Globe and Mail* editorial of December 3, 1991, the writer says: "Governments must look for ways of increasing incentives and reducing costs." He goes on to say: "Alternative delivery systems, such as community health organizations, where salaried doctors can earn bonuses for keeping patients out of hospital, should be tried more widely." And finally: "Hospitals that want costly new equipment should be encouraged to finance it by earning a surplus on their budget." [6] What has this person been smoking!

Ask any community health centre (CHC) physician employee about the likelihood of reducing hospitalizations by practising in a CHC. Ask any physician or nonphysician CHC employee about the likelihood of earning a bonus from any government-sponsored CHC. You have a better chance of winning the jackpot at the lottery. Ask any hospital manager about the likelihood of ending up with a budgetary surplus let alone financing new equipment out of same? The word bonus is not a common part of government vocabulary. It certainly would be a welcome addition if such measures were built in to the system, but they will be long in coming.

Ideas that Should be Considered

We need to make the reader understand that almost any measure a doctor takes to save the health system money (at present) is ultimately likely to be at the doctor's expense. This is the main reason why change has been so difficult. Decreasing direct patient services reduces income. Explaining to patients why something is not necessary takes much more time than dashing off a prescription, or ticking off items on a lab requisition. Alternatively, decreasing the indirect costs of allied services (e.g. lab tests) definitely saves money. This area requires attention, and a number of ideas have been put forward, most of which have not been implemented.

According to Professor Jane Fulton, Health Policy Analyst at the University of Ottawa, Canada has excess healthcare capacity as a result of health planners in 1964 miscalculating that our population would be 37 million today. We are ten million people short of this projection. Thus we have, according to some, but not all experts, too many doctors. An editorial in the *Globe and Mail* of December 9, 1991 addresses this.[7] The question then is what to do about too many doctors and too many hospital beds if one believes this is the problem. The Barer-Stoddart Report favours an immediate 10% reduction in medical school admissions. It would take a while for the ripple effect to actually save the system money. As will be discussed later in the book, the Association of Canadian Medical Schools has a very detailed manpower report in absolute opposition to Barer-Stoddart's conclusions. Who can we believe?

In private industry, excess capacity is handled by employee lay-offs. Alternatively, many senior white collar staff, especially in government, are encouraged to retire early with generous financial incentives. However, doctors are self-employed for the most part and that eliminates these strategies. As many as 25% are salaried, however, and thus potentially subject to early retirement strategies. Other initiatives might be directed at doctors to voluntarily (with some incentive) give up practice, take a long sabbatical, or change directions.

A very simple strategy to save BOTH doctor service fees and associated test services costs could be to pay the doctor not to practice! Call it an early retirement severance package, pensioning-off or whatever, some kind of innovative incentive plan to move doctors out of practice. Since many doctors have not planned very well for retirement, they keep working because they can't afford to quit. By removing a doctor from regular practice one removes both annual income from direct patient services and indirect laboratory and other test costs to the system. This proposal might not be taken seriously, but it could potentially save a huge amount of money. A bit more complex in today's rights-oriented environment could be forced retirement at age 65.

If provincial health administrators cannot swallow such an outrageous proposal as paying a doctor not to work even if it saved money, how about limiting the medical license of such redirected doctors to a new designation such as advisory or informational medical officer? Then the government gets its moneys worth by setting up in business such contractually paid doctors who are interested in participating. They would be available on a regular basis as health advisors to help the public with a multiplicity of aspects relating to their health or preventive activities. Such health advisors might be very advantageously used in starting a campaign directed at both the public and doctors as to methods for reducing health system abuse and waste – a health resources conservation corps. An entire new direction – informational medicine – is possible in such a scenario.

In a sense, Community Health Centres are a potential vehicle for accomplishing the above-mentioned idea, but to date it has not worked. The main limitation of most Canadian CHC's is that the doctors working in them generate large external patient test cost components in their regular operations. If a way of globally-budgeting the test component could also be accomplished, there might be considerable savings. Part of the reason this has not materialized to date in Canada is that laboratory, and other tests are usually provided by diverse and fragmented commercial subcontractors not under the same roof. There are many diverse sources to potentially negotiate with, and annual loads are hard to anticipate. Canadian CHCs in my experience have had little if any in-house lab, scanning or other diagnostic equipment to do other than the simplest of tests without external referral.

Of interest, in an attempt to correct this CHC equipment insufficiency, and to try and motivate the Swedish public to seek more first contact medical care at the general practice level, the Swedes have recently started a major initiative to make community health centers more attractive than alternatives (consultant, emergency department, etc.). First they have initiated the differential user's fee mentioned above. Next is a plan to re-equip CHCs with most of the diagnostic tools they will need to be equally as attractive as the hospitals. Thus, laboratory blood analyzers, ultrasound, and other equipment previously only available at hospitals, will be used by primary care doctors to better serve their patient populations closer to home. This will be a bonanza for manufacturers. It remains to be seen how much money will be saved. Easy access and proximity may further proliferate testing!

It has also been proposed and rejected that each doctor be assigned an annual block of money for tests, and this could be proportional to the last years total. To act as an incentive to reduce tests, the doctor gets to keep all the money left at the end of the year as a bonus for husbanding such lab resources. The reader will immediately exclaim, hey, the doctors won't order any tests and will keep it all! Although that is highly unlikely, there is the possibility the swing might be too far to the minimization of testing. If this idea has merit, let the government and the doctors sit down and simply negotiate what kind of formula might be devised to make such an idea work.

A less complex management problem than the block payment, would be an annual bonus to those physicians whose total yearly test cost component was lower than average. Given the computer systems most provincial health ministries use to keep track of services, it should not be particularly difficult to come up with a formula for rewarding doctors for practising exemplary cost-effective care.

Approaching a system in which limits are being imposed (government officials favour predictable annual health budgets as opposed to unpredictable and uncontrolled growth), a physician that says no to a patient request for some service, be it a test, a note excusing absence when it is questionably valid, an unnecessary prescription, should be perceived as a hero, not an uncooperative or unsympathetic doctor. How to create such a drastic reversal in public perception is truly challenging.

Refuse Payment for Sick Notes

Health costs incurred by patients seeking sick notes/certificates, could be abolished instantly by requiring such visits be paid for by the patient or his/her employer, or by employers not requiring such certificates. Such notes are in fact the doctor acting as an agent for the employee at the expense of the government health plan, validating absence when most of the time, the doctor was not in attendance at the time of the illness. In Britain, in the early 1970s, it was estimated that 50% of all doctor patient encounters were specifically for the purpose of obtaining such notes!

Pay for Telephone Advice

Doctors are constantly being asked on the telephone by patients (as a convenience), to diagnose and/or prescribe medications or arrange tests or appointments with other physicians without seeing the physician for a formal visit. It is not uncommon for these requests to come from patients who have not been seen for extended intervals. The public has become very concerned with convenience and it is often inconvenient to the employer to excuse an employee from work. This is consumerism, part of the paradigm shift. It is quite a public relations challenge to deal with such requests without offending. We are expected to minimize office visits on the one hand to address the overservicing critics, and to deal effectively with patient concerns on the other. Every time medical associations propose a new fee-schedule code for telephone advice, the health ministry administrators throw up their hands in horror, reminding us that we are overpaid in the first place, and that such professional telephone time is part of regular fees. Finally, they admonish us that such a code would be the most abused fee in medical history. These lines of argument, of course, go a long way to improving declining morale.

Thus, more and more doctors have lately forced patients to come in for appointments after any telephone request. It may be naive to believe that fewer office visit fees would result if an alternative, less expensive telephone advice fee existed, but it's worth consideration. Or, maybe the government might just make a flat payment for patients annually to cover this and other miscellaneous items. Currently, some doctors do just this, the so-called administration fee. Regardless, doctors can expect to receive increasing telephone requests for attention from the public.

Finally, I return to a recommendation earlier in the book about rewarding doctors and other health professionals for attempting to educate patients about wasteful visits and services. Consider a new fee code, "unnecessary visit counselling service." This could be a standard lecture about the lack of any need for seeing a doctor for colds, flus etc. The ministries of health might even develop an entire kit which could be used for this. A video tape, or tapes, might be created to educate patients about the folly of taking antibiotics for viral illnesses, and so forth? Perhaps this could be part of a larger program that would include public service ads and programs on Public Television? We do it for AIDS awareness and drinking and driving.

Proposed:
A Health-Cost Reduction Motivational Research Organization

I need not remind you that suggestion boxes in most Canadian work environments tend to be somewhat dusty. Most employees ignore them. The Japanese, however, have been very successful in encouraging their workforces to take an active part in their zero defect manufacturing practices. I refer to a *Globe and Mail Report on Business* magazine item in March 1992.[8] Even in Canada, Japanese companies have been able to mobilize the creative suggestive capacity of their workers. How did they do it? At CAMI, a General Motors-Suzuki joint venture in Ingersoll, Ontario, employees accumulate points for each suggestion they make and redeem them to purchase goods from Consumers Distributing catalogue – 55 points for every $10 worth of goods. Year-end awards are worth up to $1,000 each and, in 1991, 17% of the plant's employees qualified for an award. CAMI workers are coming up with an average of 4.9 suggestions per person per month. The focus of the suggestion system is on small improvements workers can make themselves. President Masayuki Ikuma tells employees, "We are not looking for home runs, we are looking for base hits."

If we are going to get our Canadian medical house in order, we need everyone's input – hospitals, clinics, nursing homes, offices, drugstores, public health centres – everywhere people interact with our health system. I hate to say it, but material rewards or recognition seem to work. We have to provide real incentives for improvements. Perhaps an area with much potential would be to set up some kind of Health Cost Reduction Motivational Research Organization for saving healthcare dollars. Such an institution would solicit any cost-saving ideas, no matter how offbeat, from both the public and health professionals and reward good or implemented ideas with recognition of some kind, possibly along the lines of the above-mentioned model. Maybe a bonus or royalty if the economic impact of the idea was significant. Such an organization could fund cost-saving experiments throughout the health system at many levels and regularly publish or promote truly useful techniques. The present atmosphere in the health system is not conducive to such spontaneous contributions. The grass roots healthcare provider does not feel disposed to do much, nor does the public. Everyone seems to be content to let government or academics have all the ideas.

CHAPTER 7

REFORM, INNOVATION: IS IT POSSIBLE, WANTED, OR LIKELY?

Predictable Government Reactions

The provinces have just started to review the recommendations of British Columbia's recent Royal Commission (ah yes, another one!) on Health Care and Costs. Its 400-page report, *Closer to Home*, contains 359 recommendations for change. The head of the commission, B.C. Court of Appeal Justice Peter Seaton, confirmed (happily) what has been already mentioned in this book, that, in the province's health system, it is bureaucracy and entrenched attitudes that kill initiative and stifle change. That's putting it mildly!

The report goes on, not so happily, to recommend things which are totally contradictory. It is in favour of entrenching in B.C. law the five principles of Medicare: universality, accessibility, comprehensiveness, portability, and public administration. This will supposedly end threats to Medicare such as extra-billing, hospital user fees and a two-tiered system. On the one hand, Justice Seaton notes the stifling effect of a bureaucracy, and on the other hand, he proposes to cast the bureaucracy legally in stone. And he expects initiative, innovation, and change from the participants? An absolute government health monopoly will NEVER achieve the health system changes his report recommends. He has not recognized the irreversible process of change underway. He offers more of the same: a more centralized system, lacking adaptiveness, competition, incentives, telling people what to do. Only the telling is now going to be closer to home.

Some of the Closer-To-Home recommendations are:

- Move healthcare out of hospitals and into peoples' homes and communities, resulting in a 25% reduction in hospital beds;

- Restrict the province's doctor supply;
- Impose an annual global cap on payments to doctors;
- Monitor billing practices and conduct regular audits of doctors' billings;
- Increase welfare rates for families with children;
- Initiate a province-wide school lunch program;
- Refuse entry to immigrants testing positive for infectious, incurable disease;
- Impose mandatory AIDS tests for pregnant women, healthcare staff and patients undergoing medical procedures in hospital;
- Permit euthanasia and death with dignity;
- Entrench in B.C. law the five principles of Medicare to end threats to Medicare such as extra-billing, hospital user fees and a two-tiered system.

Articles in *The Globe and Mail*, November 18, 1991, cite examples of what is likely to happen anywhere a government tries to run the system too closely: "150,000-strong march across Paris yesterday to denounce a growing "crisis" in the French healthcare system.... Doctors, pharmacists, dentists, nurses and other health care workers staged one of the biggest demonstrations seen in France over the last 10 years..."[1]

The French Medicare system is close to collapse, and many health jobs are unfilled. The situation is growing worse as government creates an atmosphere so uncomfortable as to drive young people away from health careers as an option. The principal complaints appear to be against tightly controlled economic policy, poor working conditions, low pay, and a critical shortage of nurses:

"We have become like factory workers," said Ms. Hauswald, 31.... "More often than not we just administer what is medically necessary for the patient. For example, if a baby is crying of pain we don't have time for soothing words," she said. "We have to continuously move on from one patient to the next..."

The crisis in French nursing has been brewing for years.... Nursing schools, unable to recruit students are faced with empty classrooms. One expert noted recently that at the current low rate of enrollment, the number of nursing schools could be reduced from 318 to 150.

Hospitals, in turn, are trying desperately to fill thousands of nursing positions that remain vacant year after year.

> "There is nothing attractive about the profession any more for prospective students," said Professor Jean Laugier, vice-president of France's university hospitals and chairman of three teaching hospitals in Tours, 220 kilometres southwest of Paris. "It's a low-paying job that entails long work hours, including some weekends, and it doesn't allow for much of a family life . . . ."
>
> The starting salary for a nurse is about $1,300 a month . . . . the best [one] can hope for upon retirement is $2,000 to $2,200 a month . . . .
>
> "As much as you like your job, after a while you really become desperate when you are faced with such working conditions," [Jean Francois Pont, 29, pediatric intensive care nurse at Hopital de Clocheville].
>
> "The question is: are we willing to invest more in our healthcare system?" [Prof. Laugier] The answer for now from the government appears negative.
>
> Already many nursing graduates, discouraged by the bleak prospect of a career in France, are crossing the border to Switzerland. The French government, for its part, plays down the seriousness of the situation, claiming that hospitals should be able to do more with less.[2]

The French government has also have missed the message of the paradigm shift. This shift not only affects consumer behaviour, it also affects healthcare workers. They will not tolerate poor conditions when they themselves have become consumers. Why should modern healthcare workers be expected to live out the old Florence Nightingale image of the nurse as totally dedicated, self-denying, long-suffering, menial, ever altruistic?

Innovation: Is it Wanted?

As the financial crisis deepens across Canada, increasingly one hears the call to arms from politicians about efficiency and new ideas and initiatives from hospitals and doctors for saving money. These motherhood suggestions are hard to disagree with, but past history does not give this writer much to be optimistic about. Innovation? Initiative? Let us look at a few examples.

But first, a disclaimer! The author is neither in favour nor opposed to the following examples of medical entrepreneurship. Whether the services are good or bad, fulfill market needs, or are exploitative, is up to the reader to decide. What is instructive from these examples is how very negative the atmosphere is for health system entrepreneurs and innovators in Canada, and how unlikely change will be if Canadians do not start to see how our attitudes are killing initiative.

The Housecall Adventure, as I shall call it, is an example from Ontario, but the scenario could have been repeated in other provinces. The public has complained for many years that as medicine has become more sophisticated, services such as the venerable housecall have gradually become unavailable. There are many good reasons for the decline of such visits. Doctors used to be among the few people in town with transportation. Telephones were few. Now everyone has telephones and wheels. In the old days, the housecall and the home were the primary locus of the doctors' attentions to patients' concerns. Doctors carried most of what medicine had to offer in their black bags. Such visits were as much pastoral as therapeutic. Medical science's entire diagnostic repertoire was contained in the doctor's eyes, ears, hands, and stethoscope. Today, most support services and/or diagnostic tools are available only in the hospital, office, or clinic where we can more precisely diagnose some of the illnesses precipitating requests for housecalls. However, this is not the point of the anecdote.

Most would argue that support, comfort, reassurance, and occasionally direct medical treatment, are sufficient justification for housecalls. Most family doctors still do housecalls on selected cases, mostly as pastoral visits for regular patients, often the elderly. However, more than ten years ago a few enterprising physicians and other business people, sensing an unfulfilled market need, set up Physician Replacement or Doctor's Replacement Services, specifically designed to fill the enlarging gap left by lack of medical coverage on evenings and weekends. This was to grow into a predominantly housecall service business utilizing moonlighting intern and resident doctors. This was primarily an urban phenomenon.

For a number of years everyone seemed to be satisfied with such operations. The regular physicians were on call less often as a result of replacement services' coverage, and got to spend more time with their families (a growing trend). The low-paid interns and residents had an additional source of income and an opportunity to gain real world practice experience. Then, suddenly, in 1990, the managers/bureaucrats at OHIP (Ontario Health Insurance Program) took notice that the numbers of services with housecall service codes in the medical fee schedule were beginning to take off as additional house-call service entrepreneurs realized there was room for more than just a few competitors in this seemingly untapped market. It may be that the OHIP computers had not previously been able to zero in on service code activity levels.

Provincial Health Ministry Surveillance Systems

The particular OHIP software program currently performing this surveillance function is called The Physician Monitoring System (PMS). This huge computer program constructs statistical models based on many factors including physician age, alma mater, practice location, specialty, availability of hospital beds, and teaching affiliation. The model predicts incomes and billing patterns and compares them to what is actually billed. In this way it can blow the whistle on physicians who deviate significantly from its norms.

The PMS pinpoints physicians demonstrating extraordinary activity out of the vast mass of physician billing data. A more detailed audit can be done for those doctors flagged by the PMS. Such audits are conducted using the Physician Profile System (PPS). OHIP officials think of the PMS as the filter and the PPS as the microscope.

The new Ontario Health Insurance Number (HIN) cards will allow tighter scrutiny and tracking, not only of doctor activities, but patient usage. Ontario patients have never before been targeted for what may be unwelcome attention by the OHIP computers and officials. The even more powerful monitoring systems in development will make it relatively easy to single out and send warnings to over-utilizing hypochondriacs as well as hyperactive doctors!

Back to the housecall story. Now, if a service will send a doctor over to my house or apartment, absolutely free, for problems ranging from head colds to headaches, insomnia, renewal of birth control pills, hangovers, not to mention serious illness, after hours, this is a much better deal than Pizza Pizza's weekly special! Occasionally drug addicts even manage to fool naive housecall physicians into renewing lost prescriptions for pain pills, or prescribing new prescriptions for their migraines. As even more entrepreneurs got on the housecall service bandwagon, the managers at the ministry of health, now downright alarmed by computer housecall service code usage trends, decided to make some changes.

Unilateral Government Moves

In 1990, the managers at OHIP unilaterally slashed payments for housecall service codes billed by any housecall service doctor. The original fee would still be in effect for visits by a patient's regular physician. Outraged, a group of housecall service business people launched a lawsuit against the Ministry of Health and to their absolute shock and disbelief actually won! (Few lawsuits against government ever succeed.) The judge ordered OHIP to reinstitute the original fees, and to pay back the lost billings due the housecall services, over $1 million. An appeal of this decision by OHIP also lost. The lesson to the Ministry of Health was simply that OHIP managers do not have the authority to arbitrarily devaluate or eliminate service code payments just because they don't like what is going on. Such authority resides in negotiated agreements between OMA representatives and government officials.

And so, the housecall service goes merrily on, It is difficult to know whether this is a patient-led or a doctor-led abuse of the system, where it is an abuse. We all know, however, that many fewer visits would occur if people personally had to pay out-of-pocket for the convenience.

The point of this example is that in our current system, any effort by providers to be innovative, either within the current fixed-fee structure or outside of it, and however altruistic or mercenary, if the innovation costs money, it is vulnerable to being squelched by unilateral government action.

The message is that doctors are free to innovate, but if they succeed, the rug may pulled out from under them. They might not be as lucky as the housecall doctors. Most doctors, or medical entrepreneurs, have understood the message loud and clear. The government will punish anyone too successful at accommodating the public's sense of entitlement in healthcare. Any innovations will be by government initiatives.

Health care innovations resulting in increased patient demand and increased costs are simply not wanted. In a rationing environment, anything that happens to service increased demand gets shut down.

It will be harder for the government to shut down the now burgeoning Walk-in Clinic phenomenon, but you can be certain they will try. Making health services too accessible is just not good for the already financially strained health plans. The fact that many of the visits to walk-in clinics are for very minor complaints and often represent convenience visits more than real medical problems, is certainly a valid concern. As well, many of these "service encounters" are duplicated by follow-up visits to the patient's family doctor. That there are too many frivolous visits to doctors in general is not in dispute. What is in dispute is how to deal with them.

Finally, a short piece appeared in *The Globe and Mail*, October 3, 1991, about another unilateral move by the Ontario government to stop paying physicians delivering hair removal or electrolysis services.[3] It seems some observant and enterprising physicians, both dermatologists and general practitioners, discovered a rarely-used service code, Z121, epilation, some time ago, and set up clinics to capitalize on it. Annual payments for this code zoomed from $16,000 in 1984 to $11,000,000 in 1990!

Once again, the innovators (health ministry officials view such hustlers as opportunists to be policed) have been put out of business. Since very few doctors were making a killing on this code, their departure from the electrolysis business will not likely result in a law suit. Ontario Ministry of Health officials learned from the previous housecall experience. This time they made all the correct legal moves, and obtained public and medical association support for the service termination. Needless to say, the traditional non-physician electrologists, also voters, and greatly outnumbering the medicos, were delighted with the government action. If you happen to be a woman with a true hormone problem causing heavy secondary body and/or facial hair, you are out of luck for any cosmetic epilation treatment as this is now no longer a benefit of Ontario's health plan.

These reactions from government directed to innovators guarantee that fewer and fewer doctors are likely in future to try and do anything requiring the slightest imagination, for personal or public benefit. **If finding and succeeding at innovation is next to impossible in Canadian healthcare where profit is the motivation, can you imagine how likely health professionals are to come up with cost saving innovations for the system when loss of income is the incentive?** As things stand, it seems only government will initiate health service ideas, and these ideas tend towards doctors being legislated into practicing the way the government wants.

A typical example of government-supported health innovation is the Ontario Ministry of Health's Health Innovation Program, funding at great expense a women's clinic in downtown Toronto. That's not to say that I don't believe such a service will be very much used and appreciated by women. But can a clinic to compete with the province's physicians, many female, who are already servicing the female population fairly well according to most opinion polls, be considered a true innovation?

The public has heard again and again in the news over the past year about Canadians being sent to the U.S. for drug and alcohol rehabilitation at a cost to tax payers of hundreds of millions of dollars. One highly-publicized patient incurred costs of almost $500,000 for treatment. Additionally, patients are sent to Buffalo to have their kidney stones blasted (extracorporeal shock wave lithotripsy) due to underfunding of such treatment locally. Similar situations occurred for patients requiring heart surgery. There are countless stories of such out-of-country payments because local doctors could not get funding for local facilities.

To be sure, the government has now put the lid on some of the more outrageous practices, but where is the public outrage at the attitudes that drove some of our best practitioners out of Canada and killed home-grown innovations or initiatives?

While federal and provincial governments may be trying to kickstart Canadian business people in general into a more competitive and innovative mode, such attitudes do not appear to be wanted in the healthcare sector. The message to date is that, *"entrepreneurs are not wanted in any area touching the health industry."* This seems incredibly short-sighted given that economists consider healthcare as one of the few potential areas of opportunity in the New Economy of the '90's. Some very clever and innovative Canadian health professionals have been totally discouraged by this attitude. This is Canada's loss. The passage in 1984 of the Canada Health Act, federally prohibiting extra-billing, and followed by similar provincial bills in the next few years (Bill 194 in Ontario in 1986), together with overwhelming government opposition to medical innovators, has not encouraged medical entrepreneurship.

Further Barriers to Change and Reform

Canadian health policy planners have been resolute in resisting any health system reform that includes both public and private sector health systems operating in parallel. Why is this so? Times change, new approaches are necessary. Many other countries, including Sweden, are now doing an about face in their attitudes to market-oriented healthcare. Great Britain, Germany, and Australia are seeming to be able to live with compromise.

The philosophy espoused by Canadian defenders of this policy is that any alternatives in the private sector favour the wealthy over the poor and thus are undemocratic. Thus, at present, the philosophy of "Less for all predominates." It seems to me there is an equally strong argument to be made that it is undemocratic to deny alternatives to those who want to provide services to those citizens who are prepared to pay for them.

In fact, alternatives already exist for the so-called non-benefit services of Cosmetic Surgery and Nursing Home Care. If you are prepared to pay up front for plastic surgery in Canada, it is available, rapidly and of high quality. Thus the poor must remain undemocratically unshapely, but the better-off are allowed to improve their appearances. In fact, extra health services will always be available for those willing to pay, and to cross-border shop! But to benefit, our service providers must seemingly also go south.

Another anecdote from this author's five-year experience working at a Community Health Centre in an economically depressed area of Toronto, demonstrates the impossibility of controlling access to desired services. No fewer than eight women, living on social welfare, came in requesting referral to cosmetic surgeons for mammoplasty (surgery to increase breast size by breast implants). In spite of their economic circumstances, or an attempt by their doctors to dissuade them, not one of these patients had too much difficulty finding the then (1975) up-front fee of $1000 for the operation.

In the *Toronto Star*, November 17, 1991, a long article in the Insight Section entitled "The Hospital Squeeze," outlined the drastic measures under consideration by the Ontario Ministry of Health. One possibility was that a 70-year-old might not qualify for a triple bypass heart operation. This particular comment provoked some strong reactions, and one of the most powerful was by Dr. Susan Lenkei-Kerwin, Cardiologist and Director, Inpatient Services, Cardiology Division, The Toronto Hospital, whose letter in the December 2, 1991 *Toronto Star* (quoted with permission) follows:

> In the November 17 story, "The Hospital Squeeze" you report that the health ministry says triple bypass operations may no longer be performed on 70 year olds. Health Minister Frances Lankin should reflect on the fact that these citizens have served their country faithfully over many decades. Some of them are World War II veterans. It was their taxes and their contribution to Canadian society that made the current healthcare system possible.
>
> The majority of these senior citizens lead an active and productive life, much more so than a number of younger peo-

ple who have destroyed their lives with excessive smoking, drinking and drug abuse at the expense of society. The health minister should look at the senior segment of society with kindness and consideration. These citizens should be treated with the respect and compassion due them.

Aortocoronary bypass surgery is a well-established procedure to improve both the quality of life and longevity. The frequency with which it is performed here is less than in other developed countries, indeed less than that recommended by the World Health Organization, and less than one-third of that performed in the U.S.

Even in the unlikely (but not impossible) scenario where age becomes a treatment determinant, does this also mean that should this person be prepared to pay for heart surgery out-of-pocket, that he/she be denied this possibility as well in Canada? And, if such a patient is allowed to buy the triple by-pass in Canada, does this put him at the front or back of the line? If the health policy planners decide to deny this hypothetical 70-year-old (the thin edge of the wedge in denying services) access to Canadian cardiovascular surgeons, and this patient chooses to go to the U.S. for the operation and give them $80,000 instead of keeping their patient's $30,000 (less than half the U.S. cost) in Canada's system, it seems like cutting off your nose to spite your face! Our health system, which is being forced to close facilities and lay people off, can not afford to lose this income. Also perplexing in this is the question, "If such a patient is denied this procedure in Canada due to being over the age limit, and has it done in the U.S., will provincial health ministries subsidize the American health system at the rate they would have paid for the identical procedure in Canada?" Why send the business south?

In the *Globe and Mail*, November 17, 1991, on the same day as the above mentioned article appeared, there was an interesting article on a recent memo from Manitoba Deputy Health Minister Frank Maynard, discussing some limited services his province should be selling to sick Americans (or others). The proposal, as one might expect, has caused a firestorm of political controversy. Manitoba health economist Michael Lloyd cited as an example the University Hospital, in London, Ontario, where approximately 20% of the open heart operations are performed on cash-paying Americans. Mr. Lloyd also said that those who argue that sick Canadians would be shoved to the end of the elective surgery lists in favour of cash-paying Americans forget that hospital beds might never be created (or kept open) if it were not for the potential cash boon brought by non-resident patients. Why shouldn't we be earning "export dollars" with our healthcare expertise? Especially when we are said to have *excess* capacity in staff and facilities?

Reform?

So where does this leave us? Our citizens and government urgently need to broaden their view of what a health system represents. Healthcare, and the activities of such a complex human endeavor, offer unlimited opportunities as part of the New Economy. This author believes it is essential for the future of Canadian healthcare to construct some kind of system that offers the public more options than they have currently. Somewhere between the excesses and deficiencies of the American health system, and the fiscal difficulties in Canada, must lie ways and means to provide essential care services to all Canadians, but also provide an atmosphere much more conducive to the creative and entrepreneurial energies of those Canadians who want to create alternatives. If we cannot resolve this problem, our health system is doomed to a inevitable descent into mediocrity.

Worse than mediocrity, the failure to attract, tap, and sustain Canadian creative and entrepreneurial energy within the health system will end up losing such talents. The wealth and jobs such enterprise generates will follow these essential, rare and restless spirits to the U.S. or elsewhere.

CHAPTER 8

WHAT ARE OUR GOVERNMENTS UP TO?

Although hospitals all over the country have been in a constant squeeze financially for years, nowhere is this situation closer to crisis proportions than in Ontario. Ontario hospitals receive about $8 billion per year for operations. Daily the newspapers deplore the $200 million deficit accumulated by more than half of the province's 220 hospitals. As previously mentioned, St. Michael's Hospital in Toronto, at $63 million in December 1991, had the largest single debt. These deficits are not a new phenomenon, and we have all heard of government bail-outs of previous hospital debts.

What is new this year is deepening fiscal constraint, with governments insisting that there will be no bail-outs. The Ontario Ministry of Health has devised a strategic plan to de-emphasize the expensive centralized institutions (hospitals) in favour of the less expensive (many question this) and more community-oriented health centres and home care. The likely ramifications of this strategy are not only that many hospitals will have to close more beds and lay off further staff, but some, possibly thirty, hospitals will be closed totally.

Even if there are excellent and convincing logistical and economic arguments for eliminating specific hospitals, it is still politically a very dangerous manoeuvre. A community will lose its hospital after all, with the convenience and reassurance that entails, and it will lose jobs and related income. Dennis Timbrell, a previous Tory minister of health for Ontario, and now the president of the Ontario Hospital Association, is demanding that the health ministry be more specific about its plans to decentralize care and de-emphasize hospitals.

It is much too early to ascertain the cost-saving potential of this shift as the Community Health Centre program (CHC) and Ontario's Health Services Organization (HSOs) are not presently in a position to replace very much of the hospital-based system of care. Most CHC/HSOs are small, with only a few doctors, and with none of the facilities or depth of support necessary to perform other than the simplest medical interventions. Such facilities have few of the sophisticated diagnostic tools available in hospitals.

Who Should be Going to Emergency?

Most hospitals, in addition to delivering complex and expensive surgical care, provide less sophisticated ambulatory care to patients in emergency and outpatient department clinics (OPDs). Here, specialists and general physicians provide follow-up care to patients previously hospitalized or seen at the emergency department, say for a cast removal. Many critics maintain that such hospital-based services cost much more than the equivalent services in outside doctors' offices or clinics. Reasons given are that hospital-based doctors tend to do more expensive tests, and that more intra-clinic referrals occur for chasing after esoteric medical diagnoses rarely confirmed. Access to costly imaging and other high technology services at hospitals also may make it easier to do an unnecessary brain MRI for a headache patient.

Thus, some experts believe ALL OPD services should be abolished and shifted to outside doctors who tend to run leaner medical practices, and provide less costly care. As well, most care is delivered with fewer staff, as these facilities, not subject to the staffing rules of the nurses' unions, simply employ fewer or no nurses. This has happened in many U.S. hospitals.

Emergency rooms (ERs) are a commonly abused resource. Patients who present themselves to the ER staff believe they have an emergency. Most experts in medicine who have studied this problem agree that, conservatively, less than 20% of all cases seen in such facilities are appropriate for emergency treatment. Some would say less than 10%. Whichever of the two figures one likes, there are a lot of services being delivered in emergencies that could be more appropriately handled by other health facilities. The term "could" is used because this is an ideal. People use the emergency department as it has become a path of least resistance to care: it's convenient; they can't get in touch with their regular doctor; they are not in their home town, etc. The list goes on. Many of these arguments are perfectly reasonable. The average family doctor is neither available 24 hours a day, nor weekends, nor is he/she likely ever to be available all the time to handle these less serious problems. Increasingly, doctors simply are not prepared to sacrifice family and health, and always be on call like the fictional old-time doctor of the movies and television. Perhaps HSOs or CHCs will evolve to fulfill this role, but we're a long way from there yet. Walk-in clinics have also not as yet evolved to fulfill or replace the emergency department.

There is a more complex explanation for the growing use and abuse of emergency departments. It has its origin in the growing fragmentation of healthcare generally. In the past twenty years, general and family physicians have gradually been squeezed out or removed themselves voluntarily from their previous close relationship with the hospital. As more and more specialists became available, and the competition for a limited number of beds in the hospital heated up, the hospital has become the domain of specialists. This is particularly true in city hospitals and, since most Canadians live in cities, this is a universal problem.

There was a time, which many patients remember, when you would call your family doctor for some emergency, and he would more often than not meet you at the emergency department and deal with it personally. I remember this well because I used to do it frequently myself, even in the big city. But, gradually, this changed. As we doctors got further and further from the hospital, not only did we stop doing this, but we lost contact with those we knew in the ER, until we were no longer known by the staff there at all. Where we might have called and arranged for emergency management of a patient, now patients go directly to the ER without any intermediate step in many cases. There was a combination of benign neglect on the part of doctors, a degree of territoriality on the part of emergency departments (family doctors felt less and less welcome), and a growing consumer attitude which requires instantaneous gratification, no delays, which brought us to the current situation.

Now, interestingly, articles are appearing which indicate that the hospitals having the most problems, generally, are the ones with the least primary care physician involvement. "Communication screw-ups, sloppy co-ordination, isolated, confused patients may be the price for years of estrangement from family physicians," says a report from the Hospital Council of Metro Toronto.[1] It is clear for the future that there must be a resolution of this centrifugal syndrome (the flight of primary care doctors away from the hospital), and that the solution is reintegration and cooperation collectively throughout the entire framework of healthcare. A tremendous challenge!

The economics of hospital emergency departments are complex, and vary from city hospitals to smaller community hospitals. The trend has been for downtown teaching hospitals to pay doctors sessional fees or an hourly rate for time spent rather than fee-for-service. The emergency department usually negotiates with the health ministry an annual global budget. This is usually based on the previous year's activity or patient flow. The trick is to figure out the minimal number of staff needed to service demand without causing patient-flow backlogs, as loads on ERs are unpredictable.

Also, increasingly, ERs are being designated as to the level of critical care they can deliver. Specialized trauma centres are staffed with very well-trained critical-care teams (few general hospitals can handle the types of cases these special units treat) who do not want to see the run-of-the-mill cases. Thus, in order to attract doctors to ER practice, many smaller general hospitals pay ER physicians a fee for service. Although there are a number of payment methods, overall, there is a growing crisis attracting doctors to ER practice across Canada (in the U.S. emergency medical care is a catastrophe), particularly in smaller communities.

We can expect to see emergency departments closed increasingly and those remaining open specializing. The doctors on staff will be on salary. Salaried emergency doctors have very much less financial incentive to see patients with non-emergency problems as they are not paid on a fee-for-service basis and, thus, will more readily redirect patients elsewhere if their problems do not fit the mandate (care level) of that particular department.

Let Them Use Community Health Centres!

As a result of federal freezes on transfers to provinces in April, 1991, a number of provincial legislative initiatives have ground to a halt. In Ontario, a review of the Public Hospitals Act, scheduled for spring 1992, will probably not occur. Aspects of the Independent Health Facilities Act, particularly new licensing provisions, are stalled.

Other major legislative reviews are also underway. We mentioned that the current Ontario Health Ministry favours Community Health Service organizations. However, the entire alternative payment program for physicians, more commonly known as the Alternative Payment Program, has been under review since early 1990. All new applications have been frozen for two years during the review.

The Community Health Centre, CHC as it is commonly known, tends to be sponsored by a non-profit community group or board, and generally has a social service orientation, with or without any actual medical services. The CHC is generally funded by a global budget negotiated annually with the provincial government. All employees are paid by salary. If there are medical services, they are provided by salaried doctors. The global budget covers expenses for CHC overhead including employee salaries.

An HSO or Health Service Organization, on the other hand, can be community sponsored or physician sponsored. To date, in Ontario, the majority, but not all, of the HSOs have been physician sponsored. Payment mechanisms vary but the dominant method is a capitation agreement negotiated with the provincial government. Capitation fees are paid on the basis of a monthly per capita fee for every patient signed up (registered/rostered) with the HSO. Registration implies that the individual will obtain ALL their PRIMARY LEVEL CARE from this organization and its health professionals. If referral to secondary level care (hospital) is necessary, then such costs incurred are billed to the province on behalf of hospital and associated medical staff.

These per capita fees vary on average $10-$15 per rostered patient per month. The actual capitation payment is age-dependent and has been based on provincial average fee-for-service rates which take into account OMA fees and general doctor-patient encounter costs. Thus, for example, an HSO with 2000 patients rostered would generate (depending on average age of the rostered patients) $200,000 to $300,000 per year for the HSO totally. From this amount the HSO would pay rent, salaries, equipment, disposables, etc. Formulas can be quite complex and arrangements within the HSO for gross income distribution are up to the sponsors to decide. Note that in capitation-type settings, the government pays the full amount whether any patients are seen by doctors or not. That is why it is called capitation. However, the HSO is obliged to keep their rostered patients very happy because if they seek healthcare anywhere else the HSO pays a penalty. Any patient receiving primary care from a non-HSO physician, clinic, hospital, etc. results in the cost of such external encounters being subtracted (negation rate) from future HSO payments to the clinic.

There has been a lot of controversy about CHCs, HSOs and health maintenance organizations (called HMOs in both Canada, the U.S. and Britain). While many Canadian health economists and ministry planners seem to feel HSOs will save a lot of money, a growing literature in the U.S. and Britain attests to the folly of this thinking. [2] American HMO/HSO costs have been rising as fast or faster than regular fee-for-service costs, and many American HMOs have gone bust. The reader should know that while most Canadian HSOs have been very limited in scale in terms of numbers of doctors, nurses and other allied health professionals, with several exceptions (Oshawa, Fort Francis and Sault St. Marie clinics), American HMOs are generally very large and employ hundreds of staff and occupy large and expensive facilities which in many cases include hospitals. In effect the American HMO models are really regional insurance plan systems.

In Ontario, CHC/HSO policies particularly penalize practices in urban ghettos as the capture of patients by the HSO is never complete. Even although a patient signs on the CHC/HSO roster (and thus is not supposed to obtain primary level healthcare from anywhere else but that CHC/HSO they are rostered with) such patients do in fact get primary care elsewhere. Thus, large penalties (the negation rate) can accrue to clinics in these poor areas of cities where substance abuse (drug, alcohol) and other social problems result in subscribers seeking care where they can get what they want, if the HSO doesn't (from the patients viewpoint) cooperate. If my HSO doctor (correctly) denies me tranquilizers or narcotics, I'll go elsewhere to get it.

The author worked in such a centre, Springhurst Community Health Centre, a community-sponsored (board of directors), capitation-based HSO in a poor inner city area of Toronto called Parkdale from 1972-1976. It became apparent early in our community health centre experience that, in spite of this clinic being a teaching satellite of the Toronto Western Hospital Family Practice Department, we would go broke very shortly due to the uncontrollable non-HSO service encounter chargebacks (negation rate) accrued by patients visiting competing doctors in the same locale.

In fact, down the hall in the same building in which Springhurst operated its clinic, there was a physician (known to the city police and the RCMP) doling out prescriptions for pain-killers and tranquilizers at the rate of almost 10,000 pills per month, practising his unscrupulous style of medicine for the entire time we operated in this neighbourhood. This doctor was eventually prosecuted and had his license to practice withdrawn. We only learned most of this much later.

Spring's Story

Slipping into the first person for a moment, I'll relate an interesting and not atypical anecdote about a patient I remember well. Let's call her Spring. Spring first came to me at the Springhurst Community Health

Centre in 1972. She was complaining of a swelling in the neck and general ill-health. After a careful history, a physical examination and a few blood tests, it was quite apparent that she had hypothyroidism, or underfunctioning of the thyroid gland. The thyroid secretes the thyroid hormone which is central to an individual's metabolic level. Additionally, I suspected she abused tranquilizers, but we did not focus on this initially. I referred her to an endocrinologist at The Toronto Western Hospital, where she was easily stabilized on a small amount of regular synthetic thyroid hormone, Synthroid, taken as a single pill, once per day.

For the next few months Spring was quite compliant, taking her medications regularly and visiting our clinic for the required follow-up and monitoring blood tests. I came to know Spring quite well, and as she learned to trust me more, we started to deal with her Valium dependency which had varied from 15 to 20 mg per day for many years. She never had any trouble keeping her supply assured from any one of several neighbourhood doctors.

Over the course of the next year with great reluctance, Spring was able to reduce her Valium habit to less than 5 mg per day. I once referred her to the Addiction Research Foundation in Toronto, but she did not stay there long. She seemed to be doing quite well, and looked and felt much better than she had for years.

I lost contact with Spring about 15 months after she first arrived at Springhurst. Then, almost three years later in 1975, looking much as she had when I first met her, Spring returned to our clinic, because she was unwell, and on this occasion, suffering lower abdominal pain. I asked where she had been, whether or not she had been taking her thyroid hormone, and was she taking more Valium again? She answered, yes, she was taking the two medications. I inquired into who had been prescribing both these medications and she was quite elusive, but indicated some neighbourhood doctors.

My examination indicated her current abdominal pain was an acute pelvic inflammatory condition. An elevated white blood cell count confirmed this. Her pelvic infection responded well to antibiotics and ten days later she was much better. When I asked Spring, "Why did you come back to see me after all this time, rather than one of the other doctors you see so much more often for your medication refills?" she answered simply, "Oh, Dr. Weiss, I go to the other doctors to get my drugs, I only come to you when I'm sick." I suppose this should have made me feel better, but it just saddened me. I never saw Spring again, but I often thought about her.

After five hard years there, my associates and I decided to leave our community health centre. Our earnest attempts at preventive medicine had fallen on deaf ears. Our monthly clinic days, on which we would talk about topics of general public interest, and have tea and cake following, were only sporadically attended. We employed several nurse practitioners to provide some primary level care, and preventive health counseling, but likewise, they had marginal success. It had become very obvious we were fighting a losing battle with the HSO concept in this district. Patients like Spring, and others, who viewed us as only occasionally necessary, were inadvertently leading us to insolvency as a result of their (unenforceable by our HSO) visits to other doctors.

In spite of frequent attempts, by both the doctors in our clinic and the local community directors, to persuade administrators at the Ministry of Health HSO Program that perhaps their funding formula should make allowances for the social problems specific to Parkdale, we were never able to get the charge-back formula modified in any way. But one of the other major difficulties we encountered at Springhurst, in our annual contract negotiations with the Ministry of Health, was a constant changing of rules!

Health Service Organizations, Revisited

Most HSO programs assume that doctors seeking alternative global budgets have already established a viable practice in terms of numbers of patients (belonging to) registered with the physician/s, or an annual budget could not be estimated and negotiated with government. That doesn't help idealistic young doctors starting their careers. There is very little reason for a doctor with a thriving fee-for-service practice to switch.

Another criticism this author levels against such alternative payment programs is that they have not been proven to be any more cost-effective than fee-for-service methods, and in fact growing studies confirm that in the U.S.A. their costs are rising as fast as regular caregivers. HSOs and CHCs are subject to facilities legislation. Such legislation often spells out the number and types of staff necessary for regular operation. One explanation why HSOs are more expensive, mentioned earlier, is that they must use more nurses than private medical facilities and thus are subject to nursing union rates and required staffing. Also, in spite of academics arguing that HSO doctors have more time to spend per patient (not being on the fee-for-service treadmill), in fact many salaried HSO physicians have been found to spend more time at committee meetings and other non-patient management activities than fee-for-service physicians. HSOs are not a panacea or the Ontario government would not have frozen the program.

It is no secret the Ontario ministry's goals for the HSO program have not been met. The program has not increased peoples' involvement in health promotion and wellness programs, a desired goal, and it has not promoted the increased involvement of allied health professions in the delivery of routine family care.

Ontario's HSO-salaried physicians reacted with alarm recently when they received a letter from the Deputy Minister of Health, Michael Decter, serving notice that their contracts with the ministry would be terminated in six months (April 17, 1992). According to the ministry, under the new agreement between the government and the Ontario Medical Association, the OMA has attained the status as the sole negotiator for all the doctors in the province. Because existing contracts are between the ministry and individual doctors or group practices, it is not possible to transfer the contracts over to the OMA. This is just one more very good reason that many are speculating that the whole HSO program may be on its way to the dumper.

Expected as part of the new NDP government's hard-line, in their review of the HSO program, is an increase in the negation rate. In the ministry document, "New Beginnings," it is proposed that an HSO not only be docked the negation amount, but the full cost to OHIP of paying for an HSO patient service incurred outside the HSO. In the U.S. the problem is kept under control by making people pay themselves for encounters outside their designated HSO.

The per capita payment for each HSO patient on the roster has previously been based on provincial average fee-for-service billings. "New Beginnings" is questioning this basis for per capita payments and would like to lower it. There has been the suggestion that these tough moves are yet another deliberate attempt by government to phase out the entire HSO program because it has not served up to expected cost-savings.

Even if the HSO program continues in a slightly or even a radically different form, the reader must be reminded that an HSO (at least most of the Canadian HSO models to date) is neither a hospital, nor is it an emergency department. The types of problem such a facility will be allowed to treat should be very carefully outlined in its contract agreement. HSOs were never intended to replace the full service capabilities of a hospital. One of Canada's major problems, and the subject of some criticism in the U.S., is that while the Canadian healthcare system is great at dealing with colds and sniffles in terms of access to health professionals (even though most such visits are unnecessary), our system falls down badly in delivering rapid solutions to more complex, institutional-based problems.

Restricting Out-of-Country Health Plan Payments

On October 1, 1991, the Ontario Ministry of Health stopped their previous policy of reimbursing Canadians for all medical costs incurred while visiting or living in the USA and other countries. They will still pay for such claims at the Ontario equivalent service code rate. The shortfall for hospital day rates could routinely be $500-$1000 per day (U.S. funds) while hospitalized, and many other services (doctors' fees, tests), could result in patients with no supplementary insurance owing American health facilities many thousands of extra dollars. It was expected that most other provinces will follow suit soon (Alberta has now done so). This is a significant change for over 1.3 million Ontario citizens. Over 500,000 Quebec residents winter in the southern U.S. This public/private shift in care doesn't seem to bother the doctrinaire proponents of universal publicly-funded Medicare!

This move has created a bonanza for travel insurance companies. Most offer health plans with escape clauses refusing coverage to those over 65 with *prior medical conditions* treated or controlled by drugs. If you can afford Florida, you can afford the insurance, our governments say. When these companies have more exposure to the actual costs, we can expect their rates will soar! There may be, as well, a bonanza for doctors, since there will soon be a lot of documentation needed for travel insurance applications, especially documenting *prior medical conditions*, and it will end up requiring patients to visit their doctors for follow-up, letters, and reports – on the provincial plan.

What Price Consultation? Caps and Clawbacks!

The recent deal between Ontario's NDP government and the OMA is the first in a rash of expected joint ventures between government and physicians to begin the task of finding cost-controlling and cost-effective measures for saving Medicare.

Under the terms of this agreement the OMA has gained binding arbitration, recognition as the medical professions' official bargaining agent, and a voice in recommending how cost-cutting measures should be brought in.

The Ontario government succeeded in negotiating caps on physician incomes. Doctors billing between $400,000 and $450,000 will only receive two-thirds of the amount over $400,000. Doctors billing over $450,000 will only collect one-third of the amount over $450,000. The reader should be reminded that very few doctors in Ontario currently gross this sum. There is the perception (fostered by some) that most doctors are making this kind of money but, for the great bulk of us (sadly), it just ain't so! It is estimated that fewer than 4% of Ontario doctors are affected by this cap, mostly specialists.

Additionally, the OMA negotiated a complex cost-sharing agreement that included a little known (by the public), and widely-disliked "clawback" formula which will result in the profession as a whole being held 50% responsible for annual cost "overruns" from "excess utilization." Typically, then, if doctors collectively exceed an agreed-upon total annual services' cost, the profession will have to pay back the difference. That has in fact happened in fiscal 1991, and the overrun was about $70 million. Thus, doctors will have to collectively share this with government and pay back $35 million. Salaried doctors are exempt; only fee-for-service doctors are involved in this formula.

In 1991 doctors collectively had total billings of 11% more than the previous year. The agreement called for only a 7.6% increase. The excess is 11%-7.6% or 3.4% (50% of 3.4 = 1.7%). Thus, 20,000 Ontario doctors must pay back $35 million or 1.7% of their previous annual earnings. The exact method is yet to be determined.

There has been much discussion recently amongst grass-roots doctors about this clawback. Many do not feel the equal burden of the payback is fair. They maintain there is no incentive for individuals to keep to the budgeted increase. Thus, for example, Dr. Doe, who bills the same as the year before, pays the same percentage penalty as another colleague who doubled his billings! Yes, increased billings result in more clawback for the higher earner, but the principle of the equal percentage penalty irks many physicians. According to the OMA, it wrestled endlessly with this before deciding on the equal clause. Reasons given include the fact that doctors may increase billings simply because they had more work to do, which was not voluntary. If the hospital was busier one year, hospital-based radiologists and anaesthetists have more work to do overall. Since this is beyond their control, must they be penalized? The clawback issue will continue to be hotly debated.

Additionally, under the agreement, physicians and government officials will be asked to find ways to deliver cost-effective medicine, and make recommendations about the controversial issues of the supply and distribution of physicians. Thus, the Joint Management Committee has met several times to formulate a plan. Four "Domains" have been targeted for top priority.[3] The First Domain, the care and maintenance of the agreement, will be handled largely by a technical committee. The Second Domain is physician resources. The Third and Fourth Domains are technology assessment and optimal practice patterns. To address such a large agenda, a freestanding, arms-length institute has been proposed and funding sought. Without the economic clout of a solidly-established organization as proposed, it would be difficult to implement identified practice guidelines. All of this is going to take a lot of time and money.

Privatization: The Double Standard

Speaking about the recent B.C. Royal Commission On Health Care and Costs report, Chairman Mr. Justice Peter Seaton of the B.C. Court of Appeals, who served as chairman of the commission, in a telephone interview by *The Medical Post*, said, "Overall, reducing services and shrinking government involvement may mean development of a private [healthcare] sector. I sure hope it doesn't come down to the rich getting better services."[4] This kind of comment is most puzzling. The rich already do get more if not better services. What else is new? For government to contain government involvement in healthcare, those services excluded must officially become the domain of the private sector. That is the point of the exercise! Cosmetic surgery already provides for this. So do nursing home accommodations. There is a basic rate the government pays and a co-payment the patient or their families pay. There is quite a range of nursing-home accommodation in Canada, from sparse at the low end, to sumptuous at the high end. And whereas an average citizen requesting an annual physical on the plan gets a varying assessment from doctor to doctor, if a senior corporate executive has his company pay privately for his annual Executive Assessment or Health Screen, the executive gets more physician time and attention, including more laboratory tests and imaging as part of this assessment. Finally, those who can afford it, and don't feel the local health system panders to them sufficiently, simply fly down to some fancy medical centre in the U.S.

Do Salaries for Doctors Save Money?

When healthcare administrators (and socialists) gather to plan the containment of the doctors (a common preoccupation), a favourite topic is whether or not fee-for-service payment should be replaced with salaries for doctors. The horror of fee-for-service for a health system manager is its openendedness. In this situation, annual budgets can never be predicted let alone adhered to. Salaries are predictable, manageable. However, some salaried physicians tend not to be highly motivated to deliver large volumes of service. Perhaps this is the ultimate goal, an indirect method of rationing? The recent *Barer-Stoddart Report*, commissioned by Canada's deputy ministers of health, along with 52 other recommendations, believes salaries and caps are essential in more specialty and primary care areas.[5] What is always remarkable to me is that ministry of health administrators always remorselessly attempt to monitor salaried CHC and HSO doctors, to make certain they are earning their keep, by counting the number of patients they service, in much the same way the fee-for-service doctor is monitored. Those salaried doctors not matching the productivity of their fee-for-service counterparts are considered slackers! It truly makes one wonder.

The doctors who choose CHC/HSO practice partly do so because they hope to be able to free themselves from the burden of being on a piece-work treadmill; this is one of its principle attractions. They also believe they will be able to better keep up with medical advances by more reading and continuing medical education courses. As well, HSO doctors, perhaps more collegial than their solo fee-for-service counterparts, tend to get involved in more committee activities. Practising preventive medicine takes time and also results in lower patient volumes. But, when they do all this, they are judged as falling short in patient service. These doctors are penalized for doing the very things that HSOs are supposed to do. No matter what health ministry people say to challenge such allegations, this is an accurate description of their attitudes.

In the much-praised CHC and HSO system of care, it has been assumed that salaried doctors, freed from their workaholic ways, would be able to spend more time with patients, and thus emphasize preventive aspects of health. This has not happened in fifteen years of the HSO programs in spite of very earnest attempts by at least some of the HSOs. That is one of the reasons the entire program has been under review. Why is it then more likely in the future? While Dr. Michael Rachlis, in his book, *Second Opinion*, believes that talking prevention is great, and that it will save the health system billions, he recommends (on page 303) that doctors who choose to practice preventive medicine should be paid less than regular doctors!

Reduce the Numbers of Doctors!

This is one of those ideas that have been floating around for as long as most remember, but somehow, no one ever gets around to actually implementing them. Money will be saved if the number of doctors is decreased by closing and/or downsizing medical schools and stopping immigration of doctors from other countries. To be sure, some steps have been taken recently. The *Barer-Stodart Report* called for a 10% reduction in all medical school classes, and governments look like they will implement this recommendation. Some medical schools have already made reductions in the number of applicants accepted. We keep hearing that doctor immigration has also been curtailed, but there is little evidence of this.

What is constant in all this manpower analysis is that no matter what the oversupply of doctors, provincially or nationally, excess medical capacity never results in a solution to the maldistribution of doctors. They just keep flocking to the big cities. No one has yet conceived of incentives which are strong enough to induce doctors to confront the difficulties that small-town and rural practices impose. Economic incentives don't appear to do it, or the amounts offered to date have not been sufficient to encourage it. The facts are very clear. Fewer and fewer general surgeons, anaesthetists, and general practitioners are going to under-serviced areas. Even the Draconian measures of Quebec's health ministry have been ineffective. There, and recently in Ontario, it has been proposed that doctors choosing to practice in cities receive much less for the identical service code fees they would receive if they set up practice in a smaller community. Quebec's measures have been quite effective in getting doctors to move . . . but it has been out of the province to the U.S. or Ontario![6]

Most senior doctors doubt the wisdom of sending, as has often been suggested, inexperienced young doctors to the boondocks as a kind of medical Peace Corps. Isolated and overworked, many lack not only the support of their more experienced colleagues but also many of the tools that doctors in urban areas take for granted.

You might wonder at this point, why the government has not placed all the doctors on salary long before now? The doctors are wondering the same thing, since it has been their chronic fear for years. One possible explanation has been rumoured amongst doctors for almost as long. The anecdote goes something like this: Once, some years ago, when the health ministry planners had had it up to here with the doctors, they commissioned a study on the subject of "Putting All the Doctors on Salary," by some nameless management consulting company. It was fully expected that the exercise would result in a relatively simple strategy to launch such a program in a reasonable time frame. However, according to rumour, the study turned up the totally unpredicted fact that, if all the doctors were put on salary, we would need THREE TIMES as many doctors to deliver current levels of service! It is also rumoured that the government has repeated this exercise more than once (with different consultants), with the identical conclusion. It makes a great story, whether it is true or not, and so it continues to circulate!

Recently a 40-page report appeared from The Association of Canadian Medical Colleges (ACMC) that completely disagrees with the *Barer-Stoddart Report* and suggests we will see severe doctor shortages, beginning in ten years, due to a number of factors.[7] Dr. T. J. Murray, dean of Dalhousie University Medical School and president of the ACMC, said that, "The *Barer-Stoddart Report* did not provide data (substantiating the need for a reduction), but said it was a societal decision without providing any further clarification."

The ACMC maintains that many specialists (particularly surgeons and anesthetists) are reaching retirement age and will not be replaced in sufficient numbers. Also, as previously noted, young doctors and women doctors in particular, have significantly different practice patterns than older doctors and will not be available in sufficient numbers to deliver the care the rapidly aging population will need. As well, reliance on foreign doctors' immigration is unreliable as they tend to distribute themselves exactly as do Canadian graduates, mostly in urban areas.

Some Twists on the User Fee Theme

In Canada, next to proposing we join the United States as the 51st state or abolishing Medicare, personal responsibility for health benefits received is the worst eventuality conceivable. However, critical times demand drastic measures. By introducing some kind of tax for health services utilized by an individual on an annual basis we would simultaneously be creating personal awareness of usage, and an incentive to utilize healthcare resources prudently. Critics will point out immediately that taxing unavoidable health service utilization is unfair, and that taxing only discretionary usage would be rational. We probably all concede this point. However, monitoring discretionary usage is harder to implement, and who is to be charged with validating the specific circumstances? Additionally, when a patient knows that each medical test associated with health encounters is also taxable, there is much more incentive (theoretically) to both patient and doctor to select very carefully which testing alternatives might be pursued.

Quebec is now considering such a measure. One idea proposed to deal with unavoidable health services vs. discretionary services is to tax the first $2,000 worth of health services utilized as part of taxable income.[8] This would be similar to a deductible in an insurance policy. Since costs much beyond $2,000 would likely be related to more essential and uncontrollable health costs (serious illness), this group of patients is protected. Such a tax however would only raise about $400 million per year in Quebec. Such a tax would overcome some of the problems associated with a user fee, such as its collection costs and violation of the Canada Health Act. It would be relatively cheap to administer, as the billing data resides within the health ministry computers, and users would just receive a tax slip each year.[9]

The Quebec Federation of Labour reacted quickly to Health Minister Marc-Yvan Côté's proposals by charging the government was bent on penalizing sick people. As has been repeatedly emphasized in this book, the paradigm shift is resulting in growing numbers of not-so-sick people utilizing the health system. Comments like this are inflammatory, nonproductive and ridiculous! A graduated income tax on healthcare services utilized is a penalty on sick people, and also a penalty on the not-so-sick, but mainly it is a penalty on those with the ability to pay. So let's try and be fair to the really sick, and apply a motivation for restraint to the others.

The Medical Funds Account

An alternative scheme that is somewhat more controversial, interestingly, has been implemented in Singapore. Annually, each citizen has 6% of his/her income set aside (deducted from salary) by the employer in trust, in a special medical funds account, where neither government nor the person can access this money. Each time the person receives medical services, tests, etc., the payment amount for each health service utilized is deducted from this medical funds account. Additionally, a user fee is also required for each medical service. The citizen is very careful how he/she uses up this fund, as the remainder plus interest is returned to them upon retirement! Thus, if nothing is used in a lifetime, the full balance is returned plus interest in addition to other unrelated pensions. If some were used, only the remainder plus interest is returned. A twist on the good old RRSP, this seems to me a very strong incentive to a healthy lifestyle.

CHAPTER 9

REACTIONS TO A SYSTEM IN DECLINE

"Given this general climate, it is no wonder that the morale of so many practising physicians and the enthusiasm of so many young people for careers in medicine are flagging." Shattuck Lecture, Arnold Relman, Editor, *New England Journal of Medicine,* 1991

One of the principal reasons for writing this book was my very great concern for the declining morale of the health professions generally. The winds of change are howling throughout organizations of every kind worldwide, shaking loose old dictatorial and pyramidal management structures, pushing us towards a more participatory and democratic style of operation. These changes seek to involve and empower workers at every level to view their individual contributions as essential to the survival and prospering of the corporate whole. Meanwhile, healthcare systems continue to plan and make changes often with minimal involvement of those most affected by these changes.

In medical papers and journals there are increasing numbers of references to declining or poor morale amongst medical and other health professionals. Such references are not only to be found in the medical newspapers and journals, but are becoming common in the popular press. While there are always malcontents in any profession, this malaise is becoming much more broadly based and even international in scope. There appears to be a siege mentality settling over the profession.

Brain Drain

The ramifications of declines in the quality of service in the Canadian healthcare system will be very serious in the next decade. In some provinces such as Quebec, Newfoundland, and New Brunswick, serious doctor migrations out of province could cause not only greater shortages of specialists in outlying regions, but also a rapidly deteriorating educational structure at many medical schools. As of 1991, it was calculated that some 500 Canadian physicians leave for the U.S. every year, mostly needed specialists. Recent loosening of criteria for physician immigration has made it very much easier for Canadian doctors to move to and get licensed in the U.S.

More importantly, changes in U.S. Medicare payments that took effect on January 1, 1992, resulted in significant increases in payments for many primary care service codes and for reductions in many specialty codes, thus making family and general practice very much more remunerative and attractive than previously. These changes reflect the American government's changing view that the nation's health system could be improved by fostering personalized preventive care at the primary care levels.

There is also recent feedback from U.S. medical staff search organizations that increasing numbers of Canadian doctors have been responding to their mailings and regional seminars.

The evidence that morale is having an impact on patient care is now so strong that this subject deserves attention. Some specialties are gradually being abandoned (Neurosurgery, Obstetrics and Gynaecology, General Surgery, General Internal Medicine, Neonatology), while others are chronically short-staffed (Anaesthesia). Regular deliveries by family doctors are in deep decline. In Ontario, the Ministry of Health Underserviced Area Program has a chronic problem attracting medical and non-medical personnel to rural not to mention remote areas. There is no solution to this problem as yet, and other provinces have similar difficulties in spite of a widely perceived excess over-all of medical manpower.

In some specialties, fear of litigation is eliminating the regular treatment of complex cases due to the high risk of unsatisfactory outcomes. Neurosurgery and Obstetrics are the specialties within which this is most problematic. Last year one-third of all neurosurgery residents in Canada quit after one year. In many other areas of medicine the increasing frustrations of regular practice in the face of growing inadequacies in the health system take their toll. Particularly frightening is the large number of very highly trained orthopaedic surgeons that have already left and are leaving for the U.S. Almost one half of the orthopaedic surgeons have left The Toronto Hospital complex for the U.S. This is aggravated by the journals and media sent to physicians (many published in the U.S.) describing regularly new tools and products to deal with previously untreatable or unmanageable conditions, which are in short supply in Canada or completely unavailable.

Alternative Methods of Practice

What other options are open for dissatisfied doctors? Currently few drop out of practice entirely due to a need to earn a steady income. Media portrayals of all doctors as wealthy (some definitely are) not withstanding, doctors require a regular income just like everyone else. Increasingly, however, discouraged doctors are opting for salaried administrative or research jobs which remove them from the pool of available patient-care providers. This trend has been confirmed in both the U.S. and Canada. Medical administrative jobs are opening up in government and industry to act as monitors or managers of medical care: in ministries of health; Workers' Compensation Boards; occupational and corporate health; the pharmaceutical industry, etc. As salaried jobs become available in quality assurance and outcomes process areas, we will see more highly-trained care-givers moving to purely administrative roles.

Not surprisingly, and increasingly, recent medical graduates are making the decision to work in walk-in clinics or full-time locums only (doctors who act as replacements for a short time for other doctors) opting for a regular, predictable schedule that allows more time for family or other pursuits despite their probably lower incomes. Female doctors are now approaching half of all practising doctors. Most women physicians choose family or general practice and, according to recent studies, tend to practice fewer hours and do less obstetrics (deliver babies), than male counterparts. The entire concept of Family Practice, as we were taught it as recently as eight years ago, is undergoing dramatic revision today. Many doctors are creating very individual styles of practice that are at odds with the public's perception of the long-suffering doctors on the television programs who are always available and able to do everything.

Why Should We Feel Good?

What never ceases to amaze me, when one considers the current state of our health system, is the historical perspective. Doctors are being blamed for the current circumstances. Doctors never asked for universal Medicare, many strongly resisted its arrival, and ultimately, it was imposed on them. Most of the current thinking about health system solutions just seems to be more of the same: the imposition of unwanted, knee-jerk rules and regulations. Why should we feel good? It is well-known in Britain that if it had not been for the extrordinary good will and tremendous efforts of the doctors there, the system would have collapsed years ago. There is much evidence that this good will is running out rapidly in many countries.

To get a better sampling of physician attitudes and opinions, I have read doctors' letters and articles in regular newspapers, medical newspapers, and journals over the past four years, noting particularly their changing mood. I have had conversations with a wide range of physicians in many specialties, in medical schools, in intern and resident training, and in practise. When confronted with the question, "What is your perception of current physician morale, and why?" there has been considerable unanimity in their responses. I was surprised that the optimism so characteristic of the young student was tempered by a growing fear of uncontrollable changes that will limit their freedom of choice in the future. Among established doctors, general and family practitioners tend to have lower morale than specialists, viewing themselves frequently as the low man on the medical totem pole. Interestingly, and this is only an impression, family physicians in smaller communities, although working harder than some of their city counterparts, seem to be more content. Rural general practice has a much broader scope of responsibility than big city practice. There have been some arguments put forward to account for this along the line that smalltown people are more cordial, less demanding than city folk, and less likely to take frivolous problems to the doctor.

Amongst specialists there is considerably more variation. Pediatricians tend to have higher morale than many other specialists. Surgeons (procedure-oriented doctors) tend to be happier than medical specialists (non-procedure-oriented). Although high-earning specialists tend to have higher morale than others, it does not follow that high earners are all happy.

Difficulty getting patients into hospital is a growing frustration for many physicians. Many have been surprised by the drastic reduction in length-of-stays for their patients in hospitals recently, and there are glaring examples of women post-delivery being shoved out of the hospital in some cases in less than two days, and post-myocardial infarct (heart attack) patients being discharged in as little as four days. This varies from hospital to hospital. Obviously, physicians tend to reflect the morale of their specific hospital, and those institutions in severe fiscal trouble tend to have lower staff morale than hospitals seen to be in fiscal favour.

Many doctors involved in medical research and academic medicine are tremendously depressed about the declining funding available to support good quality research. Recently, fewer than one-half the qualified and excellent applications for Medical Research Council (MRC) grants have been funded. Also, not well known, is the resentment among many medical researchers of the huge and growing bite AIDS research takes out of this declining pie. We all agree that AIDS is a priority, but there are many other medical problems: Hepatitis B is just one of many other equally important areas of research. Not only researchers, but increasingly the public disease advocates, such as women breast cancer victims, also want at least as much research funding for their problem as AIDS is receiving. (In Canada in 1990, 630 people died from AIDS; the same year over 5,000 women died from breast cancer.) Many of these researchers are looking more and more to the U.S. It is not only medical research that is suffering. The longstanding underfunding of most Canadian science is a national disgrace.

Doctor-Bashing

Foremost for most respondents is the very sad observation that doctors perceive themselves as being seen to be a political problem, and an antagonist, by many health ministry employees at every level. As with the postal service, there appears to be a chronic and confrontational "them and us" atmosphere. It is almost as though physicians are grudgingly seen by the ministries of health as a chronic problem that has to be managed and that, to date, they have not been managed stiffly enough. There is very little sense of ministry employees and healthcare providers being partners on the same side. While the Ontario Medical Association (OMA) representatives happily proclaimed a new era of cooperation between doctors and government as a result of the recent agreements signed in mid-1991, there is a great discrepancy between OMA representatives' cheerful claims and the grass-roots physicians' feelings and perceptions. It would be a fair generalization to state that similar attitudes represent the relations between physicians and health ministries in most provinces. In fact, the government in British Columbia recently abrogated its new fee agreement with doctors there without consultation or discussion.

Doctor-bashing has become endemic in the Canadian media. However, recently, as journalists have been probing more deeply the multiple aspects of our current health system problems, there has been less vitriol directed at doctors per se. Interestingly, surveys have confirmed that doctor-bashing is very much more common in Canada than in the U.S.

Although critics may say this goes with the territory, many doctors have thin skins and are very troubled by this phenomenon.

More vexing than media name-calling is the growing phenomenon of actual physical violence against care-givers, both physicians and allied health professionals. There have been more actual murders of doctors in the past few years than ever before. Nurses, particularly psychiatric, nursing home nurses and case-workers, must endure growing physical abuse from patients and clients. There is a feeling amongst care-givers that they seem to have been lost in the shuffle in the public clamour for greater protection of human rights.

One hopes for interdisciplinary cooperation amongst doctors and other health professionals, but turf wars between differing health professionals increasingly feed the growing siege mentality.

Increasingly, physicians seem almost defensive and apologetic that they deliver any services at all to the public, let alone too many services. There is a pervasive feeling (more, recently) that they are seen as over-servicing patients no matter how careful they are not to do so. There is a tremendous sense of scrutiny by unfriendly, faceless health ministry administrators. There is a growing feeling that the caring part of health service is not a priority and that only cost matters anymore, and that it will always be too much.

Although doctors once believed themselves to be widely respected, this perception is fading. Whether surveys still maintain that the profession in general is still highly regarded, a growing number of doctors simply do not believe it any more. Most feel their prestige is on a one way trip, downwards.

Catch-22: High Touch or High Tech?

There also appears to be a growing anti-science and anti-high technology trend amongst the public. Currently some 20% of the public seek alternative care from a wide and growing number of non-physician practitioners at their own expense. Chiropractors will soon be recognized by the Ontario government as the fifth type of practitioner (the others are: physicians, pharmacists, dentists, and podiatrists).

A growing number of doctors are troubled by this increasing number of people seeking alternative healing. The reasons people are turning away from regular medicine, or seeking alternative healthcare in addition to regular care, are varied. The usual explanations given are that regular physicians are becoming more remote, less accessible for discussion, too high-tech, too heavily biased towards prescribing drugs, and simply doing too many tests and procedures people don't understand. Many people feel doctors are not explaining things as well as they should, not taking the time they should. The most obvious explanation is, in fact, that technological advances and change are happening so fast that doctors are actually making a generally technologically naive public fearful. Unfortunately, the gap in understanding is growing wider every day, notwithstanding all the consumerism and health-related books and magazine and newspaper articles.

ALL doctors are saddened by the overriding government concern for cost, the elimination of "unnecessary and ineffective services" at the expense of caring. Most doctors are puzzled by the fact that while the bureaucrats try to figure out how to make medical care totally scientific, and to eliminate the dread placebo effect from our interventions (the caring part of our service), sometimes, all doctors know, it is all we have to offer patients. Must the placebo effect be stripped away from medical practice, to become the province of alternative healers alone?

Low-tech, high touch, alternative care has a warm, fuzzy feeling about it. It is seen to be the antithesis of science, and promises simple solutions to existential distress. "It can't hurt, and maybe it will help," is a frequently heard comment made by many of its advocates. For the really serious stuff, we can always turn to the regular doctors. Whether such services can be judged to be effective or efficacious is another story. That such services are not being subjected to the same growing scrutiny as regular medicine is just another aggravation to doctors.

Defensive Medicine

Fear of litigation by all specialties, once a remote possibility, and a circumstance that only occurred to the bad guy doctors, can be expected much more frequently. Even though by U.S. standards our past record has been unusually light, trends are indicating that more medical litigation is occurring in Canada. Settlements by the Canadian Medical Protective Association are rising and lawyers, who have for so long waited longingly for the American lawyers' contingency fee option, may get this wish granted soon, according to a recent article in *The Globe and Mail.* The impact of such a change will increase the practice of defensive medicine, which will increase the amount of testing and documentation associated with every kind of medical care.

The recent B.C. decision in which a doctor was found negligent after one of his patients was infected with the AIDS virus through artificial insemination will fuel more defensive practices. The doctor's defense was that he could not have been expected to know back in January 1985 of the possible risk of transmitting the virus through semen. This settlement has opened up the whole issue of whether doctors should know everything in an era when this is patently impossible.

One of the growing quandaries for physicians is the problem of missing a diagnosis. Then one becomes potentially liable. This is of particular concern regarding missing the diagnosis of an early cancer. Growing public expectations of physician infallibility are unfortunately real. This attitude drives doctors to do many investigations labeled excessive or wasteful by government critics. At the same time, however, health prevention programs sponsored by government encourage patients to seek early diagnosis for cancer and heart disease, so that treatment initiated early may cure or control such problems! The alternative care world promises little, and is rarely held liable for missing something. This discrepancy in expectation and accountability is truly vexing to doctors.

Recognition for Excellence

A small excerpt from an exceptional editorial in a recent *Medical Post* by Dr. Joseph Berger echoes a sentiment widely held. The full text is in the Appendix. "Finally, of all the failings of the increasingly restrictive environment in which physicians find themselves, the most frustrating is the lack of any reward for experience and expertise in the compensation of doctors. Doctors who have grown and matured in knowledge and clinical experience after a number of years are restricted – by law – to charge exactly the same per procedure as the person who just graduated and started practice today." This rigid view of physicians as interchangeable cogs in a government machine might partially account for a documented decline in the quality of service so widely commented on recently.

Doctors at large have always known that certain specialties earned very large annual incomes, and it did not seem to bother most. Lately, as the media writes more about income caps, and the word spreads around about the extraordinarily large amounts of money some of their contemporaries have been making, downright hostility and envy are creeping in. The great majority of doctors in the past have been honest to a fault. Many doctors are terrible business people, as is well known, and previously dismissed many valid billings for out-of-province patients, for those with no OHIP or HIN number, and for numerous other situations.

As more physicians see themselves coming up very short compared to what they are hearing and reading about, they will probably not be so easygoing in their accounting practices.

To complicate this situation more, physicians feel quite powerless to do anything about improving the equation. They see their future as being worse than the present, and feel a sense of helplessness, of being trapped in unfriendly territory. They are caught between the increasingly intense scrutiny of government on the one hand, and the excessive demands of patients on the other, for the duration of their careers.

A distressing and chronic problem in healthcare is the isolation felt by many physicians. The sense of *esprit de corps* which seems so much more prevalent in, for example the educational community, seems to be missing in healthcare. Doctors neither give nor receive many strokes from each other. While tremendously supportive of their patients, they don't seem to be able to transfer this attitude to their peers and to pat each other on the back much. An atmosphere of criticism seems to dominate the social exchanges of many healthcare professionals. This is a common and unhealthy situation.

An interesting phenomenon I have observed is that physicians involved in innovation and entrepreneurial activities seem to be more optimistic than physicians generally. Not all these activities involve medicine, but most do. Some physicians actually leave medicine for nonmedical pursuits. I know of seven doctors who have left practice for unrelated occupations in the past ten years. Given the obstacles facing any kind of medical entrepreneur in Canada, it is not surprising doctors feel tremendous inequalities of opportunity compared to entrepreneurs in any other field.

Why Most Doctors Don't Want to be on the Payroll

Many health economists and health planners seem puzzled as to why doctors in general are so opposed to salaries. After all, the bureaucrats are salaried, physicists and engineers are salaried, why isn't it good enough for the doctors? How little they understand the fiercely independent nature of most physicians. It is this character attribute that has enabled medical researchers, surgeons and clinicians to spend long hours in labs and hospitals, and resulted, in part, in the medical science we collectively enjoy today.

The issue is not only money, although this is very important. **The main issue is freedom.** Most people who become doctors are intensely individualistic. Most medical students, in addition to being generally outstanding scholars academically, are altruistic, perfectionist, highly motivated, considering the chance to be master of one's own destiny to be a critical factor in choosing a medical career. Many doctors are loners. Many highly productive medical researchers spend enormous amounts of time in their laboratories, away from the daily social interactions of other employment environments. Medicine for the most part is a solo act. Yes, as medicine gets more complex, teams of professionals are involved in case management. But the old rugged individualism is still a dominant fact in the lives of most physicians. Most doctors given the choice of freedom, or the more constrained life of a salaried employee, will opt for the former. Salary implies constraint. It just is not the same. Salary implies job, and many doctors like to believe their work is more than a job.

If a day arrives when all doctors are salaried (and most doctors are very fearful of this), the quality of student that medicine attracts will be very different. Some analysts have gone so far as to say that when the dominant payment method of physicians is salary, it spells a drastic shift down in the status of the occupation to a second or third class activity; medicine is no longer a profession like law but a job. In Russia, China and most other communist or socialist societies, physicians have little or no prestige, and are on the lowest levels of the pecking order. The poor quality of these health systems largely reflects the low value placed on physicians.

Many more potential medical students in the future, with the academic qualifications required to gain admission to medical schools, will choose careers that offer greater rewards than those beginning to confront the next generations doctors. Alarming statistics support this early trend in the U.S. and Canada. Doctors are still Number One on the national incomes list. Sadly, today however, many doctors are discouraging their children from following in their footsteps.

Beyond all of these factors and concerns lies the deep sense of foreboding arising from the accelerating Paradigm Shift I described in Chapter One. Cataclysmic change is overtaking and remaking all of the previously familiar routines of all traditional professions, and medicine more than any other. We can only guess what the long term ramifications will be. In the meantime, there is little basis for optimism about future prospects for doctors in our healthcare system.

CHAPTER 10

PREVENTION: THE GREAT DECEPTION?

Does Prevention Save Money?

Prevention saves money: It seems so intuitive, such common sense, but is it? Clearly, provincial health ministries certainly seem to believe so, since they have jumped on the prevention bandwagon with a missionary zeal. Many Canadian health experts believe much of what we spend on restorative health activities could better be spent on preventive activities. Thus, to give an exaggerated example, spending $100,000 for a single lung transplant (very rare under any circumstances) is not as practical as $100,000 spent on preventing smoking. It's tough to argue with this logic. This is an unlikely scenario since smokers probably never get lung transplants, but kids with cystic fibrosis do. It's the principle that counts. Health policy shifts from treatment to prevention are under way by many jurisdictions, so inquiry as to the real benefits of such moves is imperative as it is still far from clear that prevention saves money.

Although the cost-saving expectation of prevention seems likely on the surface, it remains to be proven over the long term and we should be continually examining this strategy a lot more closely because of the ultimate ramifications in funding redirection.[1] Obviously, every youngster who wears protective eye and headgear and thus avoids an eye injury or a head or spinal injury saves the health system money, besides a lot of personal and family misery. Every cyclist not incurring head or other injuries lightens the load on treatment facilities. Every smoker and drinker who stops before chronic and irreversible damage has been self-inflicted prevents some treatment costs eventually. Fewer motor vehicle accidents save lives and healthcare costs. Drunk driving is bad; safe sex is sensible. But it is less and less easy to prevent many other chronic lifestyle and sport-related injuries.

Injuries are one thing; it is very much less clear about cost-savings in many other aspects of this very complex subject. Ironically, the hidden cost of prevention lies in raised health consciousness to the public. This is just another part of the Information Age driving health system utilization.

Longterm government planning strategies are gradually adopting a broader definition of health. Part of this overall strategy includes lifestyle promotional campaigns directed at the public which encourage dietary awareness, less substance abuse (smoking, drugs, alcohol, etc.), fitness, immunization, workplace safety, prenatal care and precautions, early diagnosis and treatment of cancer, and accident prevention. There are predictable direct costs associated with current health promotion and prevention activities. There undoubtedly will be unpredictable, unanticipated and rapidly growing future costs also associated with this strategy.

The future total costs of our health prevention programs, however, are currently impossible to estimate. Many people, having had their attention or consciousness raised by health promotion messages, go to physicians more often than they might have done previously to discuss the subject in more detail, and to be reassured they won't drop dead when they, for example, jog (something no doctor can guarantee even with much testing). Some become downright obsessive about health problems, real or imagined. As more and more prevention and health promotional messages appear in the papers and magazines, they almost always warn the reader to check with their doctor first before exercising too hard, going on a diet, etc. It is easier to do this than read a book about training protocol.

Often, entirely asymptomatic patients arrive at the doctor's office fearful of having some kind of cancer as a result of a friend or relative being recently diagnosed with same. They want a full check-up and advise their doctor to do everything possible to reassure them they do not have cancer. Others seek medical attention hoping to get the latest new cancer screening technology they read about in the newspapers or watched on television. Supportive and reassuring words and advice often simply do not placate these patients in the absence of some investigations. It is far easier and maybe even cheaper to do some investigations than to spend the time trying to explain why they are not necessary. In this example, notice the motivational dynamics at play. The doctor has more motivation to do tests than not to do them, and this is without any economic incentive, since most of the tests are done at large commercial laboratories, not by him/her.

Many people who decide to get fit overdo it and sustain injuries, from simple strains and muscle pain to fractures and damaged knees and elbows. A more extreme example of obsessive exercise is the debilitating chronic fatigue syndrome seen in many fitness fanatics, sometimes resulting in actual hospitalization! These complaints result in medical visits for treatment or reassurance. More indirect costs.

Lack of Energy, Fatigue: A Costly Diagnostic Conundrum

One of the commonest complaints patients present to their doctors is, "Doctor, I don't have any energy." They have general vague aches and pains with no focus. After taking the usual medical history and examining such individuals, clinical judgement and common sense (and statistics) would tell us most of these vague presentations are a result of general poor conditioning and/or stress. However, a growing number of patients have trouble accepting such assessments without at least some tests having been done confirming that, indeed, everything is normal. Many patients simply do not accept that such presenting symptoms can be a result of stress or poor conditioning, and search for the elusive explanation of organic illness. It seems as though people are looking for something outside themselves ("low blood," anemia or something) upon which to lay the blame.

The paradoxical thing about this is that many people will accept the above-mentioned explanation from a non-medical or alternative health practitioner (herbalist, chiropractor, naturopath, massage therapist). Medical doctors are supposed to find (and cure) objective or organic illness, not functional illness. Doctor and patient alike have become victims of their preconceived notions. Non-physician practitioners do not promise cure but healing. Our society needs to examine this issue in more depth.

Many people decide to get into prevention by going out and buying a self-help medical book in lieu of a physician visit. Some get confused by popular health books (many popular health titles have an agenda or case to be made that differs from the accepted medical view) and go to the doctor for clarification. Thus, health promotion information, like many other media activities, indirectly drives medical care demand. There are now so many health book titles to choose from on any given condition or illness that people are confused by the choices available, and while books cost in the range of $10 to $35, a visit to the doctor in Canada is still free!

The doctor is still viewed by most as a counselor whom they may consult about many "soft" things, as well as "hard" objective medical complaints and associated physical findings. If the government decides doctor visits for the purpose of information, counseling or screening are not a benefit of the medical plan, then this cost component can be controlled, but it will be difficult to monitor or manage. People will continue to buy health books, and the more they read the more they seem to want to discuss with their doctors (particularly if there are no up-front costs associated with such conversations).

We have already examined the cost ramifications of the avalanche of health information in Chapter 2. If too many people become health obsessive as a result of having their health consciousness raised (one way or another), the economic burden to provincial health budgets could be astronomical. The point to be made emphatically here is that we may not be able to prove prevention saves money, and if it does not, should preventive practices be part of the government plan rather than a choice made by individuals if they want to spend their own money on it? Perhaps government should be discussing this issue with the public?

Dr. Michael Rachlis, in his 1988 book, *Second Opinion*, as previously mentioned, believes that it is too expensive to pay doctors to play this health informing role. Perhaps he is correct? Deciding not to pay doctors for such services is a deceptively simple option for the government. So who is the best person or professional to do it, if such a role is valid? Perhaps a new job category is desired. Perhaps this is the perfect place for those surplus doctors that we might pension-off, sabaticalize or redirect at lower incomes into a new kind of role! Perhaps the overburdened school system should have this added to their busy schedule of responsibilities!

Should a nurse take it on? In this writer's opinion, in most cases there is simply too much to know. Most doctors, by virtue of preventive medicine interests and education, would probably be better equipped, if supported by information tools, which will be described in more detail in later chapters. Certainly this kind of educational task might properly be the role of a community health centre, in spite of the historical fact that such activities have so far failed to thrive in this venue. Given the right encouragement, a solid strategy, and the will, it could be done.

There is agreement amongst many medical professionals (still an article of faith) that health promotion and aggressive preventive strategies have a positive effect on many aspects of health. Many chronic illnesses are very slow in their development. Some chronic conditions are just now demonstrating evidence of potential reversal of established effect if aggressive changes in risk factor management are practised. Alternatively, some don't. Abusive lifestyles (drinking, drugs, smoking, obesity, lack of exercise, bad eating habits) definitely result in premature death and disability, but not to all. Diabetes and atherosclerotic arteries are only part of the penalty paid by the aforementioned unhealthy lifestyles.

Not so clear are the specific benefits of exercise on longevity or reduced costs at the end of life where most medical costs are incurred. Does a healthy life end in a clean, cost-free and sudden demise? Not nearly so clear. As well, how modifiable are the risks of cancer, given a genetic predisposition? This remains a very contentious issue. Increasingly, genetic factors are being shown to be crucially important to almost every human disease condition.

Does ideal control of diabetes prevent the potential longterm complications of this disease? This question has been debated for years and is currently the subject of an intensive ten-year longterm study, The Diabetes Control and Complications Trial, sponsored by the U.S. National Institute of Health. Definitive answers on this question will not emerge until at least the mid-1990s.

Much less obvious is whether the best-known multi-factorial cardiovascular risk model to date, so well pioneered and documented by the ongoing U.S. Framingham Study, can be generalized to many other disease areas. Arthritis, Alzheimer's Disease, mental illness, cancer? Can modifiable risk factors be found for these and other conditions which could prevent or delay the development of these diseases?

Many American corporations are sufficiently convinced now that preventive medicine or wellness programs reduce sick benefit payouts in the near-term that they are forcing mandatory lifestyle changes on their employees or firing those not complying. Drinkers, smokers, drug abusers, the unfit, the obese, need not apply.

This might save corporations sick benefit costs during the employment life of the employee, and thus prevent absenteeism and keep insurance costs down a bit, but does it reduce the national healthcare costs in total or in the longer run? Obviously, if I live to age 85, with never a day of illness, and drop dead, with no lengthy hospital stay for heart attack or stroke, it is cheaper than if I were to linger for a while. But what if all my running and obsessive dieting just delay my inevitable stay in hospital to an older age? What if my obsessive running causes chronic joint problems requiring some other current or future expensive treatment? There are no definitive answers to these questions yet.

Medical Screening/Preventive Medicine: How Can We Pay for It?

A frequent part of medical practice before the inception of Medicare was an assessment of how much a patient could afford to pay for services before proceeding further with diagnostic tests, etc. It was common to decide with the patient exactly what would be done, and the cost of each step, so as to get the most bang for the patient's limited number of bucks. This disappeared with the onset of Medicare, and the late 1960s were the last time Canadian doctors or patients gave any major considerations to the cost of the process, with very few exceptions.

From time to time since then, patients have come to me with an elderly parent who is visiting from out-of-country, usually a poor Carribbean island with limited medical services. Generally these patients do not arrive with any presenting or focused complaint, are basically well, and the children simply want a check-up to reassure them Mom or Dad is okay. When it is explained that there are an almost unlimited number of possible investigations, many expensive, that might be done before they could be given even guarded reassurance, we then get into a detailed discussion of what each type of screening test costs (this is the only time I ever look up the cost of tests in the *Schedule of Benefits*, Lab Section), the relative value of different screening tests, and how much is the upper limit on the cost of our screening protocol. We generally agree on a complete medical history and physical examination ($47.70), a chest X-ray ($30.43) if the patient has not had one in ten years or so (specially if a smoker), a CBC (complete blood count, $12.93), an SMA-12 blood biochemistry profile ($24.00), a urinalysis ($4.00), occasionally an electrocardiogram (EKG, $19.95) if there is any suspicion of heart problems, and settle for this minimal batch of screening tests. Total cost: $139.00 as of 1992!

Should anything come up on this screening, we then get into discussing any further measures which might be essential to clarify specific problems. This routine is certainly not exhaustive by any measure of current medical science's near-infinite numbers of tests possible. It would also not be possible to tell a family that their loved one has a complete bill of good health based on such an encounter, but that is all the patient can afford. Outside of this unusual example, there are no such pressures for Canadian doctors currently to be so prudent. The economic constraints of encounters such as the above always seemed to add a bit of challenge to an otherwise relatively routine patient-doctor encounter!

The reader might rightly ask why such economic or resource considerations do not constrain every patient encounter even today? The best answer that comes to mind is that, in the example given, the context for both doctor and patient was different. Both had clear fiscal constraints moderating the mutual decision-making.

Another similar situation, which is not uncommon currently, is encountered working in hospital emergency departments, especially those near the U.S. border, or in cottage country. An American presents some problem requiring medical attention and the patient has no insurance. Again, the doctor and patient decide on a course of action guided by fiscal constraint. Obviously, if a major medical crisis exists and the patient is not capable of participating in the dialogue because of their emergency (unconscious, severe pain, etc.), initial care is rendered as necessary.

A Philosophy of Screening from a Physician's Viewpoint

There are six generally accepted screening criteria, for use in health maintenance and screening interventions, regarding the types of screenable conditions being sought: [2]

1. The condition must have a significant effect on the quality or quantity of life;
2. Acceptable methods of treatment must be available;
3. The condition must have an asymptomatic period when detection and treatment significantly reduce mortality or morbidity;
4. Treatment of the asymptomatic phase must yield a therapeutic result superior to that obtained by delaying treatment until symptoms appear;
5. Tests that are acceptable to patients must be available at a reasonable cost to detect the condition in the asymptomatic period;
6. The incidence of the condition must be sufficient to justify the cost of screening.

These criteria are ideal guidelines which should be considered before deciding a particular "screenable disease" fits these requirements and is thus a justifiable condition to try and screen for. Rarely is this degree of rigor applied when doctors are asked by patients to chase after vague complaints.

Many patients ask me to "do some tests" to reassure them their diet has the right amount of vitamins in it. Currently most of the blood tests doctors do to accommodate these types of requests are in no way based on the logic of the previously listed criteria. Try and convince a patient who has recently paid an alternative healer hundreds of dollars for hair and fingernail analysis that these tests have no current basis or consensus in medical science!

Some Unexpected Ramifications of Prevention

A cardiological example is useful to demonstrate the kind of world we are rapidly moving towards. In the old days just a few short years ago, if you had coronary artery disease (CAD) and were symptomatic (experienced some chest or arm pain, breathlessness, decreased exercise tolerance, or heart rhythm disturbances), you had two options depending on the detailed diagnosis and characterization of the state of heart muscles and arteries. First, you took medication and continued your regular routine with some lifestyle modifications if you smoked, etc. Second, you had coronary artery bypass surgery (CABS).

Recently the waters have been muddied considerably. Consider now the concept of asymptomatic or silent cardiovascular disease (you can't feel any actual discomfort or pain, breathlessness or palpitations). In this situation neither patient nor doctor has evidence based on medical history that anything is wrong. Only more comprehensive investigation can document the presence of potential problems.

Additionally, until just several years ago, the idea of reversing, let alone arresting or preventing the progressive narrowing of patients' coronary arteries by any means other than surgery was inconceivable. Then, a number of studies including the NHLBI (National Heart, Lung and Blood Institute) Type II Coronary Intervention Trial, the Familial Atherosclerosis Treatment Study, the Cholesterol-Lowering Atherosclerosis Study (CLAS), demonstrated that mortality could be reduced, probably by some actual change in the existing vascular lesions. In addition, the International Nifedapine Trial on Anti-atherosclerotic Therapy (INTACT) study, which some feel is seriously flawed, suggested that the development of new coronary lesions (atherosclerotic plaque) could be (arrested) reduced by taking calcium-channel blockers (Adalat).

More recently, there is gathering clinical proof that aggressive lowering of cholesterol, with diet and/or cholesterol lowering agents such as lovastatin (Mevacor), seems to actually reduce the size of existing atherosclerotic lesions. It must be noted that many cardiologists still disagree with the early conclusions of such published research. As with most other medical topics in which no general consensus exists, there is much contention.

In fact, many critics do not accept today the widely held conclusions of the Framingham Study about cholesterol and heart attack risk. There is much evidence that ONLY GENETIC FACTORS are at play. Any cardiologist can cite examples of heart attack patients they have seen who had no cardiovascular risk factors at all. At a relatively young age, these patients had heart attacks or multiple coronary artery narrowings in the absence of elevated cholesterol, and high blood pressure problems: they were thin, ran fifty miles a week and so on. When asked to explain these aberrations, most shrug and simply exclaim, "genetic." Still, the facts seem to be indisputable that many patients at high risk of heart attacks may, indeed, **given the corrective manoeuvres, be able to move down the risk curve.** What are the implications of this? Probably one-third of Canadians and Americans are walking around with these types of arterial lesions and don't have any symptoms. Some of them are ripe for acute myocardial infarctions (heart attacks) depending on a number of related risk factors. Can you imagine the numbers of investigations necessary to identify and characterize ("stratify the risk" is the term used by doctors) these patients, let alone the therapeutic manoeuvres to minimize or reverse such pathology in the hope of preventing such MIs and their associated hospitalizations? The next question is how reversible is all this? Are these people all going to have MIs eventually and we are simply time-shifting the event?

As you can see, the previous discussion about the reversibility of established coronary artery narrowing, and our current inability to tell patients what their arterial status actually is without expensive and invasive procedures, like coronary angiography (a method of injecting a radiopaque dye into arteries and then taking X-ray pictures of the coronary arteries to get an image of their size), begs for a simpler and inexpensive screening method for answering this question if we are to practice really effective preventive medicine.

Recently, such a "non-invasive" screening method has been described and may be available fairly soon. The April 1992 issue of *Longevity* magazine describes the work of cardiologist Dr. Robert Lees, Director of the Massachusetts Institute of Technology's Arteriosclerosis Center in Boston.

A synthetic form of LDL-cholesterol (the bad stuff), which contains a harmless radioactive substance, has been developed that is called SP-4. When this substance is injected intravenously, it travels around the body and attaches onto areas of the arterial lining where atherosclerosis is beginning to develop and shows up on a standard X-ray film. These so-called early "plaques," can thus be identified. It is hoped this method will be able to detect the early "unstable" atherosclerotic patches which can trigger heart attacks. Early work with animals has been very successful, and it is hoped similar findings will translate to humans. If this technique becomes an acceptable medical screening technique, it is impossible to predict the popularity and economic impact of this development.

The Guideline Gap

There was much in the newspapers nationally in late 1991 about the huge cost of wasteful medical services in Canada. Cholesterol testing and cholesterol-lowering treatments seem frequently to be singled out as examples of this waste. The current and previous ministers of health in Ontario frequently note that doctors are not following the cholesterol consensus guidelines which emerged from an expert panel supervised by The Task Force on the Use and Provision of Medical Services, a joint commission co-sponsored by the Ontario Medical Association and the Ontario Ministry of Health.

This lack of adherence could suggest that family physicians across Canada are uninformed, or it could suggest that family practitioners are informed enough to maintain some skepticism about conflicting recommendations in cholesterol management from expert panels.[3] Many doctors believe it is simply too early in the evolution of our understanding about the reversibility of existing coronary arterial narrowing and the types of non-surgical treatment that should be regular guideline practice.

I predict growing confusion as the difference between American and Canadian guidelines develops. I will call this potential development, "The Guideline Gap." Because American guidelines will be developed by a medical system which will gradually become much more technically sophisticated than the constrained Canadian approach, there will, by necessity, be increasingly different standards of care for U.S. and Canadian patients with identical problems.

The controversy over cholesterol testing and treatment is a long way from being concluded. New research emerges daily which supports or refutes current positions. This is just one tiny little medical area (cholesterol, blood lipids) amongst the vast body of scientific knowledge and information involved in the regular practice of medicine. Government concern for costs, rationing measures, and downright centralized control may temporarily modify physician behaviour in the short run, but they will not change scientific facts, which emerge more slowly.

The New Genetics: The Ethical Issues of Knowing

If a serious genetic defect can be detected in utero at the earliest stages of fetal development, does the State, in the interests of costs, have the right to strongly influence the parents' decision to terminate or not to terminate such a pregnancy? Most would say definitely not. The State however might have the right to de-insure such medical situations. The parents would then have to bear the full financial burden of living with the medically predictable result of choosing not to terminate.

Take a simple example, cleft palate, a malformation of the face and palate resulting in variable degrees of facial and palate deformity. Such malformations are not life-threatening, have no long-term developmental effects and simply represent a cosmetic problem that nevertheless can be and often is disfiguring and emotionally damaging. Reconstructive surgery can repair and improve cosmetic appearance. If such a defect were preventable (by therapeutic abortion), the government could decide not to pay for all the medical attention necessary to deal with the problem. This is a very touchy area.

A more severe and life-threatening situation is Tay-Sacs neurodegenerative disease. Children born with this genetic defect are doomed to only a few years of mostly unpleasant life, and ultimate death. Medical costs are significant. This condition, however, can be screened for or detected before birth.

Mongolism is another genetic defect. Easily detected. Not so easily treated. And on it goes. How many political parties do you know that are prepared to deal with this can-of-worms? Prevention by termination in all these and other genetic defect situations could save a lot of money and misery, but who is going to draft a blanket set of legislation to deal with this increasingly detectable and preventable set of problems?

The above examples represent fairly disabling health conditions, not all necessarily lethal. We are rapidly learning to identify genes that only predispose to certain chronic illnesses which become manifest later in life. Add genes for diabetes, predilection to early heart disease, predilection for all types of cancer and particularly breast cancer, mental illness, and lately (in *The New England Journal of Medicine*, February 20, 1992) there is even evidence that osteoporosis, osteoarthritis, and abdominal aneurysm (ballooning of the artery) are gene mutation defects and we have a mountainous challenge and opportunity rising before us as a society.

CHAPTER 11

TOUGH CHOICES YOUR PROVINCIAL HEALTH MINISTRY MIGHT MAKE

Confuse the Public (and Health Professionals)

According to several unnamed Canadian cynics (many of us), there was a backroom deal to end Medicare during the Free Trade Agreement talks with the U.S., and the Prime Minister told the Americans, off-the-record, that he was planning to kill our healthcare system simply by defunding it, as he has done.[1] As well, provincial politicians are seen to have been cooperating with Ottawa's hidden plans. The deputy ministers of health have been meeting regularly over many years to change the system and their plans have little provision for public approval. Therefore, the increasing media reporting of health costs spiralling out of control is a myth propagated by the politicians to confuse the public and soften them up for drastic changes. Federal and provincial politicians have been scapegoating the healthcare system, using scare tactics about the need for fiscal restraint. Thus, the current crisis is a plot by those bent on killing the Medicare program.

Belt-Tightening Under Way as You Read This

Across Canada at this moment provincial health ministries are wrestling with a diminishing number of options, as a collision occurs between the growing demands by the public on the healthcare system and limited economic resources to pay. What follows I believe is a reasoned and fairly accurate prediction about what measures your planners are likely to take as the health system crisis deepens. Some, all, or none of the following measures might be initiated. Privatization of some aspects of healthcare, anathema just five years ago, is now being considered. The foundations of such actions will likely be strongly influenced by reports or studies like the B.C. Royal Commission Report, *Closer to Home*, and the State of Oregon catastrophic coverage recommendations.

Canada must gradually recognize that Medicare attempted to bite off more than it could chew. Globally ALL countries will gradually realize the implications of the paradigm shift underway and gradually try to extract themselves from providing more than a fraction of health products and services as this sector of the economy becomes unimaginably vast.

Blame the Care Providers to Deflect Attention

As we have seen in British Columbia, the Commission studying their health system has come out with a report which blames the doctors for squandering upwards of 25% of the annual provincial health budget on unnecessary services and procedures. Ontario was quick to follow. Quebec seems far ahead of the rest of us in harassing its medical professionals. This is not a new routine, but it seems to be relatively risk free.

Worst Case Scenario: Privatize All Medical Care Except Catastrophic Care

This is an unlikely immediate step, but one hears more and more rumours that such a drastic move is possible. Before this happens, Canadians have to decide what this catastrophic care definition means to us, and what such a health service list might comprise? The reader must also recognize that with the pace of change in what doctors can do in specific medical situations, no list can be cast in stone. Lists must be under periodic review. The precedent in Oregon is fascinating, but their choices may not be ours. The reader should know that several European countries are giving this serious consideration, and Holland, in the face of a political storm, seems to be leading the way in such reforms.

A Gentler Scenario: Make Arbitrary Cuts in Payments, Providers and Services

According to Monique Begin, Minister of National Health and Welfare, 1977-1984, in a panel discussion on CBC morning radio recently, when the Medicare planners originally projected health needs for Canada, they estimated our 1991 population would grow to 37 million instead of an actual population of 27 million. Thus, according to some analysts, in the intervening years Canada overbuilt both the health system and its facilities.

Over the next six months the reader can expect a growing PR program by both federal and provincial governments to persuade the population that since we have such overcapacity, closing some hospitals and constraining the system is not really going to jeopardize access to healthcare, but simply bring capacity in line with current population numbers.

The figure 25% is being thrown around when studies and/or commissions indicate how much waste there is in the system. The strategy is to make big cuts more palatable. What the planners back at the beginning of Medicare did not anticipate was that regardless of whether we have 25 or 37 million Canadians, the limitless pursuit of more health services per capita uses up whatever capacity is available. By the way, Canadian population trendlines appear to be accelerating recently!

If there are any lessons in history regarding overcapacity and undercapacity in terms of, for example, the cyclical supply of teachers or engineers, we can expect the healthcare pendulum to swing in much the same way. Feast or famine. We've had the healthcare feast during the 1980s, and we are entering the era of famine. As governments ramp up to decrease the number of medical school graduates, restrict physician immigration, restrict physician licensing, initiate more stringent relicensing, close hospitals and possibly medical schools, it won't hurt today; it is tomorrow (2000-2010) that we will experience the shortages. As previously noted, it's a shame the shortages will be felt at a time when the explosion in the advance of medical science is taking place.

In an article in *The Globe and Mail*, November 14, 1991, Ontario Health Minister Frances Lankin, echoing the latest B.C. Royal Commission's finding that 25% of their provincial health budget is squandered on unnecessary and wasteful activities, was quoted as saying to an audience at the Ontario Hospital Association convention, that at least 25 to 30% of everything we currently do in the healthcare system has no proven value. Sounds familiar! She called on healthcare managers to identify and eliminate this waste. She gave as an example the excessive amounts of blood cholesterol testing. Do we want to pay for cholesterol-lowering drugs for people over age 65, when the advice is that they do almost nothing to reduce their health risk? Should we continue to pay for useless treatment? The reader should not be surprised that people over 65 are expendable, in fact, increasingly we hear euthanasia touted as a great solution to the excess demand being created by older Canadians on the healthcare budget. Lankin also said, the public and the doctors must be educated.

Prevention, Cholesterol, and Blood Lipids Revisited

Let's return to the cholesterol issue for a moment. Previously in this book, we have noted the very great interest governments, health professionals, and the public have demonstrated in the role of preventive behaviours in reducing premature illness. Nowhere in medical history has such a groundswell of literature supported so extensively the value of altering blood fats (not only cholesterol) in reducing mortality and morbidity from coronary artery disease at any age. While cholesterol alone is not the only risk factor important in this disease (age, sex, height, weight, blood pressure, presence or absence of diabetes, HDL-cholesterol are also important), it is a good screening starting point. While a doctor can tell at a glance whether or not your height and weight are approximately normal, doctors can NOT guess what your blood pressure or cholesterol levels are WITHOUT ACTUALLY CHECKING OR TESTING THEM!

You cannot feel high cholesterol! You can be thin as a rail and have very high cholesterol. You can be 200 pounds overweight and have a perfectly normal cholesterol. You can have a normal cholesterol and a TOO LOW HDL-Cholesterol. Daily, patients come in to doctors' offices all over the country and, having had their "cholesterol consciousness" raised by some article or television program about health, they request the test. For all the reasons previously discussed in this book, few physicians try the, "It isn't necessary, and it costs too much" approach. One of the reasons doctors tend to repeat these tests so frequently is the variability in the accuracy of measurement; 15-25%! Add to this the fact that the values change daily (6- 8%), and that some doctors are unclear on which tests to do, and we get the current free-for-all.

On the CTV evening news, November 20, 1991, broadcaster Lloyd Robertson announced new findings in a U.S. study (Blankenhorn), that a group of patients taking Mevacor (Lovastatin), a cholesterol-lowering drug (also available in Canada), for the first time have been found to actually reverse the size of previous coronary artery narrowing as a result of taking this drug. Additionally, the same study indicated the people taking the drug had half the number of heart attacks as the group not taking Lovastatin. Once again, many cardiologists are sceptical about these findings in terms of actual lesion reduction, but there is general agreement that fewer heart attacks occurred in the test group. If this kind of insurance against heart attacks is solid, many people will insist on taking the drug for this reason alone! Such findings, (reduction in atherosclerotic plaque lesion size) have already been described by several other studies, and proposed in a popular recent book by internist, Dr. Dean Ornish, *Dr. Dean Ornish's Program For Reversing Heart Disease.* The only way to monitor such treatment is by testing cholesterol periodically and/or doing more expensive serial coronary angiography, or some other artery imaging technique. Advances in the medical treatment (non-surgical reversal) of existing arterial atherosclerotic placque can be expected to increase rapidly in the next few years. This is probably cheaper than surgical bypasses.

Faced with such studies and patient requests, doctors can comply or deny patients service. Most doctors take the path of least resistance and order the tests. If the doctor wants to deny the patient, he must be prepared to spend a significant amount of time explaining why the test is not necessary. This time will end up being charged to provincial health plans as a higher encounter fee than a simple office visit. It takes longer to say No. One way or the other it will cost money. Which is the least expensive in the long run deserves thoughtful analysis. Doctors would be happy if governments would tell patients these tests are worthless and thus will not be paid for by the plan. It would remove the onus from doctors to repeat themselves endlessly to patients.

Either we should practice preventive medicine or we should not. It is getting less clear what we should do, but the message from the government that is very clear is, "Whatever you do doctor, we don't want it to cost very much, and do your part as our cost-containment agent!"

Expect certain laboratory tests and eventually imaging procedures to be delisted. Delisting of drugs in provincial plans has already been mentioned. In Ontario, the current Drug Formulary lists about 2,500 drugs which are free for those people covered by the Drug Benefit Program (all persons over 65 and those on welfare, etc.). The government plans to reduce this list to less than 500 drug products in the near term.

Because of public concern if cholesterol testing is deleted it will not be long before it is available in malls, drug stores, doctors offices, and/or possibly self-test kits one can buy similar to pregnancy tests. This is called shifting aspects of healthcare from Medicare to the private sector or privatization.

HIN Cards and the Smartcard Health Encounter Monitoring Program

Health ministry administrators have been wrestling with how health managers can judge whether or not a typical visit to the doctor was necessary (called a service encounter in healthcare management jargon). They also want to know who initiated the service encounter, patient or doctor? What happened at the encounter, and what was the outcome? This has been a challenge since before Medicare began. Until recently, healthcare system administrators have not had the remotest idea what is going on out there. No idea whether tests or treatments are relevant or not, no idea if waste is occurring. Technology is going to make it easier to address this issue but it is going to take considerable time to get a surveillance system up and running.

By the way, you will be hearing much more about outcomes research in the future, and this is probably a worthwhile pursuit, but don't be fooled by semantics. Outcomes research is really another way of monitoring what is happening between patients and doctors to identify waste, all the while calling it "quality assurance." No doubt the reader has heard of Smartcards. If not, there has been increasing interest by health administrators recently in the potential of computer cards for tracking patient use of healthcare services. Until recently in Ontario it was impossible to trace how an individual patient interacts with the system. Bureaucrats want to know who is doing what to whom and why, and has it made any difference? The old provincial health number (the Ontario Health Insurance Program eight-digit OHIP number) was not a good enough identifier as an entire family was covered by the same number and thus it was not unique as an identifier for a single individual.

In Ontario, a ten-digit health number and Health Information Card, (an initiative of the Liberal government under Health Minister Elinor Caplan) was recently introduced. This card (similar in appearance to a creditcard) uniquely identifies you to the provincial health system computers and introduces many new quality assurance and monitoring possibilities. Now it is possible to trace your every encounter with the system, at your doctor's office, the laboratory where you go to have your unnecessary cholesterol test, the X-ray department, the hospital emergency department, etc. Any time that the HIN card is presented, another entry is made in your OHIP database file. Please note, this plastic HIN card with its little dark magnetic strip is NOT, REPEAT NOT, a Smartcard. It is no different from a credit card. The magnetic strip has very little storage capacity compared to Smartcards, and the HIN card has no computer chip in it and thus cannot do any actual computer processing by itself. The HIN plastic card is just the first temporary step towards more sophisticated and smarter cards as they become cheaper and more reliable.

The Smartcard, on the other hand, has an actual computer processor chip (the smarts) and some random access memory (RAM) on the card. This small computer chip can do more functions actively than the passive magnetic strip on an HIN or credit card. While Smartcards and other special high data storage density optical cards have had some success in France and Japan, they have not made much impact to date in North America. Ontario has been studying very limited Smartcard applications in a pilot project in Fort Frances and Windsor, but little information has been released describing how useful these studies have been. The Fort Frances Smartcard project is designed to monitor how seniors utilize pharmacy services in their community. It is unclear whether any other medical services are part of this study. Alberta also did some Smartcard pilot studies. Quebec may be further along in Smartcard experimentation than other provinces. Dubbed the *Carte-santé*, this Smartcard will contain a mini-medical file of the patient. The first pilot project started in March 1992, and includes four target groups in Rimouski, 300 kilometres north-east of Quebec City. The project is expected to last 18 months.

According to Marc St-Pierre, general director of client services at the *Régie de l'assurance-maladie du Québec*, the province's health insurance board, the primary goal of the project is to improve the quality of patient care through a better circulation of information between healthcare professionals. It is hoped the card also will reduce the useless repetition currently within the system. The four target groups, some 7,000 citizens in the study, include: seniors 60 years and older, pregnant women, newborns up to 18 months of age, and the entire population of St-Fabien, a town just outside Rimouski.

Healthcare workers having access to the cards include doctors, pharmacists, ambulance technicians, and nurses in the local community health centres and the emergency department of the Rimouski Regional Hospital. Before health professionals can gain access to a patient's card file, they will first have to insert their own access card into the computer system and punch in a personal identification number. "In terms of security, the system is nearly perfect," said St-Pierre. St-Pierre has assured critics (such as the Quebec Civil Liberties Union) that the information stored on the card will not be downloaded into a central computer bank. As well, the data on the card will not be used for resource planning.

To further ensure confidentiality of the patient file, the card's information will be divided into different zones, and most healthcare workers will have access to only those zones that concern them. Thus, pharmacists will have access to the patient identification zone and a prescription medications zone, but will not have access to the medical care zone. Physicians will be able to see a resume of the patient's medical history, the types of medications he or she has been prescribed, and the other specialists or general practitioners the patient has seen in the recent past. Certain medical conditions might be highlighted, such as diabetes or a recent heart attack. The physicians will see at a glance on the computer screen where they are in the care of this patient.

According to Dr. Augustin Roy, president of the *Corporation professionnelle des médecins du Québec* (CPMQ), his organization has no problem with the project. "The government has been extremely conservative in the design of the program," said Dr. Roy. However, it remains to be seen just how valuable the card will prove to be in the attainment of higher-quality patient care.

Optical storage cards are different from Smartcards. Smartcards have a computer processor chip on them and a varying amount of memory. Typically, a Smartcard might have between 8K bytes of RAM and 124K bytes of RAM (K = 1000, a byte is a unit of storage representing a single alphabetic character or a numeric digit, RAM stands for random access memory). While this may seem like a lot of storage, in fact, compared to the amount of memory space necessary to store even the shortest of medical histories, this type of card will not be a satisfactory portable medical record. All Smartcards are currently good for is tracking encounters and the types of service codes a patient utilizes. As well, a very brief prescription list can be stored on such cards.

The laser or optical storage card, a completely different medium, has much greater capacity, but no chip. Thus it acts only as a very compact storage place for information. The most widely tested cards from Drexler Technology in the U.S. have a capacity of up to two million bytes of storage. They utilize technology similar to musical compact disk (CD-ROM) optical storage, but the card readers are quite different from CD-ROM players, being more costly and in very limited supply. There have been optical cards rumoured to have 50 to 500 million byte or megabyte capacities, but they are still experimental, very costly, and thus impractical for wide application at present.

Monitoring Patient-Provider Service Encounters

Monitoring data from a patient-health provider encounter is a very difficult task. If it were easy it would have been done long ago. Since doctors have yet to standardize a universal, medical information recording methodology, deciding the types of data the government might want to capture at typical patient-doctor visits is a truly formidable task. Not only is there a lack of consensus amongst similar medical specialists (for example, cardiologists), but different types of doctor vary widely in the types of information they like to collect on patients. Most doctors still keep written, often illegible paper notes. While huge amounts of money have been spent over the years trying to develop standard recording techniques and formats, we are still waiting for the perfect medical record. It is likely there will eventually be specific formats for each specialty.

All doctors do agree that as the amount of transaction data they are asked to collect (on a single patient encounter) gets too large, we simply will not have time to record it. Having seen some of the proposed encounter recording formats health ministry analysts are thinking about, it seems to me likely it will take at least twice as long to enter the data as it took to see the patient! This is the ultimate barrier preventing widespread adoption of computer medical records. Many medical record data processing experts have said that until flawless and cost-effective voice-entry computer systems are developed, the aforementioned ideas are totally impractical for regular healthcare system use.

Shift More Prescription Drugs to Over-the-Counter Status

A few years ago certain antihistamines that had previously been prescription drugs were de-controlled to over-the-counter drugs (Seldane, Hismanal, Claritin). There are benefits to both patients and government from such changes. First, it is easier for the public to obtain such products as they don't need a doctor's prescription. Important to government is the cost saving incurred by reducing visits to doctors' offices for such prescriptions. It is likely that a trend will develop shifting from controlled drug to de-controlled drug as the potential economic benefits are very significant. In many other countries around the world, one can get almost any drug without a prescription. The potential for side effects and actual illness, of course, rises with the widespread use of self-medication and this could neutralize the previously mentioned savings.

Campaigns to Convince the Public Many Visits to Doctors are Unnecessary

Articles might appear in your daily newspaper subtly suggesting the best medical thinking on how many visits are reasonable for a particular health problem. Such articles will probably focus on chronic medical problems which have traditionally required recurring visits: high blood pressure; allergies; cardiovascular conditions; arthritis; psychological or emotional problems; and cancer. Following a number of newspaper articles about repeat visits, expect the next step to be restrictions on the number of visits to many different types of doctor that will be paid for. Whatever the number is, it will be less than the current unrestricted access so popular with the public. You will be allowed as many visits as you want, but you will have to pay for any exceeding the set number.

Limiting the number of visits will not only be difficult to monitor and enforce; it will create an interesting legal dilemma. While delisting a drug item or a specific type of blood test from the list of medicare benefits is relatively easy, and moves the cost to the private sector, limiting visits is tough. It means that the service code is still a benefit of Medicare and thus according to Ontario Bill 184, which prohibits doctors from extra-billing for covered services, it is currently illegal for doctors to charge patients for the service when they have used up their limit. It is not clear how this might be handled. Again, how will the government prevent a patient from going from doctor to doctor? It is fairly clear that without some kind of realtime, online transaction-based computer network none of this can be policed.

Current Services: Eliminated, Limited or Shifted to Less Expensive Personnel

Shifting doctor-performed services to alternative personnel seems to be gaining momentum. Recently, midwives have won their long-standing status fight with Ontario's government, although they have not yet negotiated Medicare fee schedules to be covered by the plan. Their fees, about $1,200 for pregnancy and delivery care, greatly exceed what doctors are paid for the same service (midwives spend more time with their patients/clients than doctors), so the cost savings side of the equation seems unlikely to pay off. However, if midwives succeed in shifting more care from doctors to themselves they may in effect shift care from hospital to home and improve prenatal care, thus saving the system money.

This is part of the reason they have succeeded in getting recognition. Nurses also have been lobbying to take over many services previously delivered by doctors. While there is no question that many services performed by doctors can be performed by nurses, what is less clear is that it will save money.

Reasons nurses might actually cost *more* than doctors include the fact that the nurses' unions have very rigid rules for how many staff must be available at a facility. These rules are very specific in hospitals. It is well known in the U.S. and Canada that shifting hospital Out Patient Department (OPD) or clinic activities to private facilities saves costs by getting around nursing union's rigid staffing regulations. Thus, the same services can be delivered in the private sector with less staff and hence cost. As well, since nurses continue to catch-up in remuneration negotiations and pay equity awards, and if they function in addition to rather than in lieu of doctors, where is the economic advantage? Also the question of midwives' and nurses' liability insurance looms as their responsibilities increase.

Shifting and limiting or delisting is a very sensitive area, and any moves will happen gradually. One can anticipate that certain types of laboratory test may be the first items shifted to the private sector. Cholesterol has already been mentioned. More likely, patients will be allowed one or more tests per year or quarter. If the number is exceeded, it becomes the patient's personal responsibility to pay for it. It will be difficult to monitor patient status unless, again, an online, realtime, transaction-based computer system is available to permit doctors, and laboratorys, other service providers to ascertain instantly what a user's situation is. Such systems do not yet exist in most provinces, although we are moving in that direction. A Smartcard system could be used to monitor this type of information, but such cards would have to be available for every patient, and card-readers at every provider office. Similar limits will be placed on other tests such as blood sugar for a diabetic.

Selfcare Encouraged

Selfcare devices have been rapidly advancing the ability of patients to measure certain medical parameters on themselves. Blood pressure devices are now quite popular and common. Diabetics are familiar with small self-test blood sugar devices. We can expect government to require patients to use these devices if they are available. Small devices that can measure a number of other blood parameters will be emerging quickly.

American companies have developed devices that can tell a diabetic what their blood sugar is without a finger puncture or a drop of blood. They work on an optical sensing principle. Selfcare has much potential, but the transition will require a lot of hand-holding.

Which types of doctor visits might be reduced initially? Logic would suggest that services viewed by health ministry managers as, unnecessary or of low priority, would fall victim early. Thus, visits to allergists and dermatologists, which might be perceived as of questionable value or to address cosmetic problems, might be axed, or severely restricted. Perhaps only those allergic problems or dermatological procedures involving skin cancer, or debilitating conditions interfering with ability to work might be permitted. It would, of course, require more extensive documentation and monitoring to police such encounters.

After all, if electrolysis services for hair removal were so easily dispensed with (Chapter 7) recently in Ontario, can moles, freckles, aging spots, spider veins and acne be far behind?

Walk-In Clinics look like a juicy target. According to health analysts, many services at such convenience clinics are of questionable necessity. So, perhaps we might decide to reduce all or some of the service code fees used at such facilities by a percentage to save money. This may or may not have any impact on patient demand, since patients like convenience, but it is guaranteed to put most operations into the fast-track to insolvency. Since few taxpayers will lose any sleep over such an eventuality, much like the collective yawn after the electrolysis operations hit the dust, the provincial health managers can potentially claim for themselves another much needed victory.

Next, general practice or family practice visits in toto would be scrutinized. Since almost half the doctors in Canada fall into this category, there is probably much fat to be trimmed here from a health manager's perspective! Again, the monitoring system is critical, and this is why there is such current interest in studying service encounters by the ministries of health. Typically, recurring visits for following patient blood pressure, allergies, diabetic status, cardiovascular problems, arthritic conditions, and emotional problems account for enormous numbers of service encounters. (See Figure 8, Chapter 6) Expect guidelines on "proper case-management" soon.

Visits to psychiatrists may come under scrutiny, and limiting numbers of sessions covered is a fairly easy way to save money here without eliminating such services. The overflow to psychiatric social workers and psychologists not covered by OHIP should be welcomed by these professionals. Patients with certain chronic diseases like lung cancer, Alzheimer's or Parkinson's disease that have no currently effective treatment may not be covered for attempts to relieve such conditions.

Force All Family Physicians Out of Fee-For-Service and on to Salaries

Measures that have been discussed so far are gentle or evolutionary. Professor Jane Fulton, Strategic Management and Health Policy, University of Ottawa, believes the open-ended and inherent unmanagability of fee-for-service will require the government to force the transition rather than wait. She predicted in May, 1992 that this confrontation will occur within a year. As well she predicts by 1993 provincial health spending will drop from the current 33% to 25% of the total provincial budget.

Dr. Arnold Relman, Editor Emeritus, *The New England Journal of Medicine* and Professor of Medicine at Harvard has long been an exponent of salaries for all doctors. In a recent two-hour television town meeting hosted by Phil Donahue, Professor Fulton invited Dr. Relman to Canada to help persuade the Canadian doctors why salaries are both desireable and inevitable. **Dr. Relman noted in this meeting that while he was in favour of salaries for doctors, he believes they should be very generous.** We all clearly understand in Canada that the definition of generous would be scaled down by 2 to 4 times, and that overtime would become common as financial pressures escalate, and that the starting salaries would likely diminish.

Details of the nature of this conversion to salaried family physicians are less clear. We have already examined the Community Health Centre issue, and while all provinces have been proclaiming the attraction that HSO medicine seems to hold for governments economically, there still appears to be ambivalence about a complete switch to this structure. The logistics of converting every physician to salary overnight is a nightmare. In order to accomplish this, the government by necessity must assign blocks of patients to each doctor. The public is not keen on such lack of choice. The registration of all these citizens is a vast undertaking. All the doctors would have to sign contracts with their health ministry. Staff numbers, overheads, and many other items, vary from region to region and even within cities. Formulas for salaries may depend on patient load, seniority and a whole host of other factors. There's no question: the administrative start-up costs, not to mention on going costs, would be immense.

CHAPTER 12

HEALTH SYSTEM WASTE MANAGEMENT

It has already been noted by the B.C. Royal Commission, and echoed by Ontario Health Minister Frances Lankin that the amount of waste in the health system has reached staggering proportions. Reiterating part of a speech recently to the Ontario Hospital Association Annual Convention, health-care experts estimate that at least 25% to 30% of everything we currently do in the healthcare system has no proven value. Unfortunately, the minister has not clarified how and where this waste is occurring. Nor have there been subsequent initiatives to identify this waste. If, in fact, wasteful activities can be identified in detail, why not selectively de-insure all such wasteful services and procedures? Is there an acceptable level of waste, as zero waste in any human collective activity is unlikely?

Health Minister Lankin then called on healthcare managers, hospitals and doctors, to identify and reduce wasteful and unnecessary services. She was less specific in identifying details of such waste and spoke more in generalities, citing a few examples where savings might be found such as: excessive diagnostic testing in general, cholesterol testing in particular, treatment of elevated cholesterol in patients over 65 years of age, in vitro fertilization, caesarean sections, too much cardiac surgery, reductions in amounts being spent on treating lung cancer and prostate cancer when it does not do much good. If we are collectively going to deal with this problem we will need more specifics and strategies, and much more time than we have.

No one from the provider side has yet responded to the Minister with the simple question, "Please tell us what the waste is and how we can reduce it." We are not certain how to do it. We wish we were. For over twenty-five years, an entire practising lifetime for most of us, we have been practising medicine in an economic cocoon. We simply do not know how to practise medicine any differently! We certainly have lost the ability to say or accept no. We do not know where to start. We are like the unfortunate Russians, Poles, East Germans, Hungarians, emerging suddenly from a centralized, state-mandated economy into the confusion of a market economy. We do not know how to be! Someone is going to have to help us. We cannot change overnight. A massive re-education program is going to be essential. A similar plea might be directed to the government from the public who are equally used to having their own way in health matters. They need as much direction as the healthcare workers. Like energy conservation in the electric power generation sector, we are being told that health services must now be looked at as a limited resource in which similar conservation measures should be taken.

Most doctors practising today were trained in an environment stressing the easy availability of a vast diagnostic technology. This led to overdependence and atrophy of some of the clinical skills possessed by an earlier generation of doctors armed only with their individual "smarts" and a stethoscope. As the detection of asymptomatic or subclinical disease, and the assurance of optimal longevity increasingly becomes modern medicines challenge, no one wants or expects a return to this more primitive stage in medical sciences evolution. High technology is here to stay whether the government likes it or not. But, if a new health resources conserver society is going to emerge from the current reforms, people must recognize that such changes will require time, patience, and much behavioral change from all the participants.

Finally, it should be noted that it is a lot easier to sit up in the ministry of health listening to experts and consultants and make grand pronouncements about how it should be, and much different down in the trenches dealing with the public. The requests that people make for unnecessary tests, referrals, etc., can, and do, overwhelm even the strongest and most idealistic resolve. Most doctors, tired of trying to reason with people simply give in to their requests because it is by far the easier path. Many patients do not want to hear reason, they do not want to hear that it isn't necessary, and the guidelines say, etc. They want what they want, and if you are not prepared to deliver it, someone else will. It would be an interesting new environment to practice in, if patients had to pay for their demands, up front, or if the health services they used annually were taxed.

Typical situations include, "Doctor, I'm here to day because my wife has bronchitis (By the way – I'm fine) and I need antibiotics (covered by my employee drug plan) so I don't catch it." You try to explain how unreasonable this request is and get a blank stare, knowing that not a word is being received because his mind was made up before you started. Or, "Doctor, I'm going away for a week and I have a cold, but I don't want it to turn into pneumonia so I came in for antibiotics." Just try and get out of it if you can! A recent and new request, "Doctor, I heard TB is making a comeback, and even though I feel great, can I have a chest X-ray?" This little sample of what our system is up against doesn't begin to illustrate the dimensions of the public's lack of knowledge about appropriate or effective measures and their desire for accommodation. If the government has a strategy for dealing with this we doctors want to hear it, preferably as soon as possible.

Some Perspectives Minimizing Unnecessary Tests

The government and the medical profession have differing views of what constitutes waste. It is important to clarify this, as nowhere in all of the thousands of words pouring from newspapers and television discussions has any doctor tried to explain the role of tests in medicine. Right up front, most doctors will agree that we do too many tests. However, some explanation and qualification is essential. Not all tests are diagnostic. Many might be classified as diagnostic, some as reassurance routines, some as motivators, some as therapeutic, some as trend indicators, some as monitors (safety, particularly in occupational and environmental medicine) some as documentors for defensive purposes, and, yes, some as placebos. Whether the government is prepared to believe it or not, there are some patients who simply will not be reassured that everything is okay until they have been told tests A, B, and C were all normal. You can discuss and explain until you are blue in the face, but the actual ritual of having blood, and/or urine taken has therapeutic value in and of itself. Is this wasteful? Unless you are blessed with magical powers, it is generally not possible to tell someone everything is okay without some physical or objective evidence to support it.

Some doctors even refer to the ordering of blood tests on people who are asymptomatic, the "worried well," (a category that covers a growing percentage of the population) as bleeding therapy, a carry-over from the 17th and 18th centuries when doctors would recommend bleeding, or leeches, as actual treatment for vague patient complaints. Such modern therapeutic bleeding, or procedure as placebo, has a venerable lineage! Doctors know most of these tests are likely to be normal, but try and tell the patient who fits the "worried well" category that everything is great and nothing more is necessary.

If some mysterious someone in government knows ahead of time which tests will be normal, and has a way of selectively de-insuring all these types of tests (making patients pay for them out of pocket?), the health system needs this input desperately. As well, we all want something to reassure the patient which would replace these wasteful routines.

We have heard from the government that much can be done to minimize such activities. What is the best way to approach this? Before any rational approach to massive waste can take place we are going to have to break this down into more manageable portions to examine each in detail. A list of what the government considers waste must be made test by test, procedure by procedure, specialty by specialty, hospital and clinic and so forth. Priorities must be set.

Until each hospital, HSO, clinic, nursing home and doctor's office can focus on what waste needs eliminating, how are we supposed to make any progress? Then having done all this, the government should have some specific ideas about how to reduce particular items. Are we to use check-list verification before a test can be authorized? It is fairly easy to override such arbitrary devices. It would be easier to have global regulations. Finally, an incentive system must be set up to reward good performance.

Government Waste

It would be a wonderful example for the rest of us, if the government could demonstrate it was also interested in minimizing waste by not squandering large amounts of money on fiascoes like the $25 million on the Royal Commission on New Reproductive Technologies, and several other recent projects.

For all their high moral and ethical principles, and great intentions, humans have a way of finding means for utilizing new and compelling technologies when governments and institutions get tied up in red tape and take too long to decide on how or whether to use something that is already useful.

Quality Assurance

In 1988, Dr. Arnold Relman, the Editor of *The New England Journal of Medicine* wrote about "Assessment and Accountability: the third revolution in medical care." The fifties and sixties were the eras of expansion, times when medical advances propelled a growth in facilities and specialties. The second phase, the revolt of the payers (insurance or government health ministries) is well under way. Medicine is now entering the third revolution, a rising interest in quality of care, an era of assessment and accountability.

Tightly intertwined with assessment and accountability are concepts of quality, notions of safety, appropriateness and effectiveness. As has been argued earlier in this book, massive information processing systems will be required to sort this out. There is great danger that the health system can become over-managed, and top heavy with administrators. Who will watch the watchers? Or is this the role of the press and the media?

Are These Services Wasteful?

We have all been watching the U.S. Food and Drug Administration try to sort out whether the current freeze on the use of silicone breast implants should remain. In Canada more than 150,000 women have had breast implants in the past twenty-five years. Many of these procedures, which the system has increasingly labeled cosmetic, are performed at their own expense, outside Medicare. If it is decided that all these operations must be repeated to remove these devices, is this to be at government expense, or personal? There is already a move afoot by one activist group demanding the government do something about all this.

Similarly, but in a much lighter vein, almost every day in Canada, someone has a tattoo removed, usually by a dermatologist, using an expensive laser machine, a highly effective technique. Should such procedures be done at government expense when the original procedure was never covered by Medicare?

Does "Managed Care" Make Sense?

The Canadian health ministers have been telling Canadians that managed care will save us huge amounts of money. The above mentioned Dr.

Arnold Relman, of Harvard Medical School, is a widely respected American physician who has written and spoken frequently on the problems of the U.S. medical system. Recently, on a network (NBC) television interview, he told David Brinkley that managed care does not save money! Whom can we believe?

He believes that ultimately the payer of healthcare costs, in Canada, the government and thus the taxpayer, must tell care providers ultimately that X, a fixed amount, is what we can afford to pay for healthcare. A fixed limit. That pretty well sets the ground rules. That is precisely where we are in Canada today, the question is, what is X? How flexible are we as a society, if, after every effort at minimizing waste, we still find out that X is not enough?

CHAPTER 13

HIGH TECH TO THE RESCUE?

"The road leading to health for all by the year 2000 passes through information." World Health Organization

Lessons From the Front Line

Distilling the experiences of over twenty years of medical practice (hospital and office-based), in both the USA (Connecticut and New York States) and Canada (Calgary and Toronto), allows me to make a number of observations. It has been very stimulating and satisfying to be able to deliver quality healthcare in Canada in an environment where cost is not a constraint to patients or to caregivers. The fact that cost has not been a consideration was both a good thing and a bad thing: usually it delivered excellent care but it totally removed fiscal responsibility and common sense from patient and doctor.

In the midst of this embarrassment of medical riches, patients and doctors alike have become too fond of, and attached to, medical tests. Partly as a result of this, and partly because of the media, there is a misperception by patients as to the usefulness of such tests in regular care. Doctors recognize lab test limitations and errors, and use tests in a complementary way, not placing too much emphasis on them in the over-all diagnostic process. Doctors understand the variability and artifacts that can occur with many blood and other tests. Patients do not have this perspective or knowledge. For most patients, putting a number on some biological parameter seems to imbue it with magical properties (for example a single blood pressure reading or even a weight). People tend to view such results far too literally, and read far more into them than the profession ever intended (some specific types of test notwithstanding). This has led the public, journalists, AND the legal profession into believing, perhaps, that medicine is more scientific than it actually is. Can we change this perception at this juncture? Would it moderate patient demand for health services? Does the government have any ideas how to modify the public's perceptions?

Before answering the last questions, consider the cosmetics industry. Many women (not all) are fairly realistic when they buy the latest lotion or potion. They know that such products are limited in their effect. Does this stop them from buying billions of dollars' worth each year? Not on your life! Many men (also not all) keep buying the latest new brand of beer even though they know it won't really make them more popular with women as the ball game advertising implies. Is the pursuit of wish fulfillment any less likely in the health field?

Canadian and American patients are identical in their demands and expectations of the health system. If anything, each year they become more knowledgeable and specific when they decide to seek attention. **The role of patient medical information-seeking must receive more attention as an engine of demand in modern health care.** Government attempts at limiting availability and access to health services and products are just going to be temporary barriers for you and me to overcome as the paradigm shifts.

Professor Glen Beck, University of Saskatchewan, commented on the TV Ontario *Between the Lines* recently, "Most people don't like going to doctors, I don't like going to doctors, they stick needles and knives into us." His antipathy to doctors was palpable. Not everyone reflects this view, or the numbers of people going to doctors would not be so high. His somewhat dated attitude (he is locked into the old paradigm) has not been the attitude of most patients in my experience of 25 years in practice. Very often many patients have nothing at all done to them in an encounter with their doctor. Not infrequently, the reason for a patient's visit is not acute illness, but fear for illness in the future, or increasingly, to find ways to enhance the quality of life and perhaps even to extend it, or to clarify some claim of extending life that they read about. A consultation may consist of a friendly chat, nothing more. Sometimes the most traumatic part of an encounter at my office is the cost of some book recommended to the patient, or an exercise routine that may result in sore muscles. Patients particularly enjoy getting health information from their doctors, and in my personal experience, preventive medicine, discussion and education are central to healthcare delivered at our offices, and it's often even taken seriously. Patients appear to like it this way.

Doctors like to be in demand, who doesn't? Doctors are happy accommodating patients, and feel uncomfortable not doing so. The government's chronic concern for costs is creating a lot of anxiety and conflict as doctors try serving two masters. People fervently wish that their doctors would listen to them and talk to them MORE! Doctors constantly wish they could do more for each patient, and don't like to have to disappoint people by not providing enough time or information at each encounter.

Almost every television health program emphasizes the important and growing role preventive activities should play. Unfortunately, this preoccupation with prevention has led the public to believe the ravages of time can be modified. It remains to be seen whether this type of practice would be available if preventive educational and counseling services were not a benefit of Medicare (not yet delisted, but a strong possibility), and only true sickness (still awaiting definition) is compensated. Patients increasingly communicate their fears about this, wondering about what kind of actual medical care will be available for them as economics increasingly dominates the medical landscape.

Unfortunately, or perhaps fortunately, fiscal responsibility is the new message. Every healthcare encounter is now suspect.

Medical Computing:
Why There (Probably) Isn't a Computer in Your Doctor's Office

Doctors have had great expectations for computers as an adjunct to care for more than twenty years. They have often been disappointed, even burned. Being chronic optimists for the most part, doctors continue to hope for the kinds of information systems that have yielded such productivity gains in science and engineering. There are many reasons why computer technology has been so slow in diffusing into the main stream of medicine (with the exception of the embedded or built-in computers in the CT and MRI imaging systems). Probably the most important reason has been a lack of coherent economic and conceptual will on the part of government and the profession and a lack of truly innovative and useful software (again, imaging and visualization software is currently a very dynamic field). The numbers of would-be medical software innovators that have tried and failed to develop the Wordperfect, or Lotus 123, of the medical world is legion. It is a very tough challenge and takes time and money, as doctors are a very tough market to convince about a really new medical tool.

Medicine is still largely a cottage industry. System-wide decision making is fragmented because each professional **individually** rather than collectively makes planning and purchasing decisions. Seventy-five percent of doctors still practice privately. We have, thus, no collective decision-making ability when it comes to system-wide planning. In Canada, only government has the power or funds to initiate large undertakings like those under discussion in this chapter and so far, it has not done so. Another more important problem is that what governments might want to achieve in health system computing, and what medical professionals might want out of medical computing, might not be the same thing.

Provincial and even national medical organizations have had limited interest in or power to effect how their membership run their office affairs, let alone their collective use of huge medical database and telecommunication systems. Few doctors have Fax machines. Currently, only slightly over half of Canadian doctors have even a single computer in their office. Most of these are used not by the physician, but by the office staff for billing. Less than 20% of this installed hardware base has the ability to telecommunicate with other computers, and little to telecommunicate about! Fewer than 5% of Canadian doctors use any type of medical software for regular clinical applications. No large system or macro decisions are possible at the micro level of the individual office. A corporate entity, capable of creating a collective will and strategy, is essential to any progress. Our governments have been very slow in showing leadership in this area. Interestingly, in Great Britain over three-quarters of all general practitioners now have their practices computerized.

Finally, and perhaps most importantly, while business and administrative professionals in non-health fields view computers as strategic tools for enhancing competitive advantage, until very recently no such essential business justification has been operative in medicine. Many businessmen have remarked in our discussions about medical computer use that since doctors appear to be able to make a very good living no matter how inefficiently they run their offices, why on earth do they need computers? Indeed, few doctors have ever been able to prove that using a computer to remit invoices to the provincial plan even paid for itself in more income, better use of time, etc. All such office billing systems seem to do is shift the monthly data entry work of the provincial plan data entry clerical staff onto our staff!

While dental professionals have aptly demonstrated the value of their billing computers to enhance income by much better recall methods for preventive dental care, calling each patient every six months, doctors have been cautioned that similar, doctor-initiated aggressive marketing techniques are not appreciated by government!

Ontario's Belated Information and Technology Strategic Plan

Only as late as April 1989, in Ontario did an Information and Technology Strategic Plan emerge from the provincial health ministry to begin to seriously utilize modern computer systems in the health system for anything more than billing and statistics. We have barely begun to develop the kind of health information systems we will need in the 1990s and beyond. Very few participants in the health system, outside the government originators, are aware of the implications of these important initiatives. Sadly, such systems tend to be planned with operational/management considerations uppermost in mind, and this is shortsighted given the possibilities of such systems as provider tools, healthcare quality assurance tools, and potentially, consumer health information tools. Hopefully, with the recent collaborative efforts between government and the medical profession such as their joint management committee, the potential of such systems will be realized. But, there is still too little involvement of the private information technology sector in health system experiments. Too few medical and health professionals are involved in these early developments. Too little joint-venturing between universities and the private sector takes place in Canada.

The Ontario Ministry of Health, and other provincial health ministries, have not encouraged health professionals to computerize until very recently. It has too long been an independent struggle by individual hospitals or physicians (early technology adopters or pioneers). The entire focus has been on computers for claims-processing only, in spite of early literature which stressed in the 1970's that this is the wrong way around. Experts in medical computing have been writing for more than a decade that billing or claims processing should be simply a by-product of the more important purpose of medical computing: the facilitation of improved patient care and the means to assure quality control and more positive and predictable patient outcomes.

Claims processing was an early target for medical computer software vendors as it is a relatively easy task to develop software for numerical applications. Billing software is really just a variation on accounting software. However, novel or innovative software developments will be necessary to make computers useful in assisting health professionals in the task of improving the quality of medical care, medical records, and other medical computer application areas. Government must help stimulate this sector, or useful software will emerge slowly or not at all. This is a very difficult and risky area (particularly in Canada where the government health system is the only market, the population is small, and each province has different needs) and the technical tools are only now emerging to make it possible. Most physicians are only minimally computer literate and have not the slightest idea what emerging or future medical software applications are needed. This potentially large software industry cries out for leadership.

Medical Records and Case Management

The capture of a paper audit trail in the regular practice of medicine has resisted every effort to improve the quality of the patient-doctor process or of *encounter information* via computers. Gradually, however, the old anecdotal notes and qualitative descriptions of findings are giving way to much more comprehensive quantitative descriptions of every medical activity. Eventually every patient-provider encounter will generate a multimedia array of digital data (text, image, etc).

Enabling hardware and software technologies that will be required to make truly useful medical records systems possible include:

- Cost-effective voice-input hardware that converts continuous speaker voice input into high quality edited computer text;
- Medical records software that can handle text, images, and sound, and integrate these diverse types of information into a coherent and easily-used system;
- Cost-effective media for storing diverse patient information, such as personal health lasercards or Smartcards;
- Powerful, large-scale (tens of thousands of users) networking systems to allow instantaneous sharing of these electronic records;
- Inexpensive card-readers to allow the wide application of these cards in hospitals, offices, nursing homes, pharmacies, etc.;
- Finally, Fax systems that can receive and convert transmitted messages into ASCII text files for inclusion in computer files; Such OCR-Fax (optical character recognition) experiments have barely started and many more should be pursued.

Areas of healthcare patient-management crying for such information-tracking experiments are: cardiology; cancer treatment; drug prescribing, dispensing, tracking and monitoring; chronic home care and other care areas where patients must make many visits to diverse caregivers. Systems that allow hospitals to support home care extensively would save millions. We Canadians can, of course, continue to do what we have always done and wait until the Americans or Japanese do it and buy it from them, but this will do nothing for our national economy and job creation. For years many technical experts have noted that Canada's health system is an ideal incubator for such new computer applications because of its logistical simplicity compared to the U.S. and because of its smaller and more manageable size. So far, however, little has been done to capitalize on such advantages.

There has been very little government encouragement or fostering of an active and vital medical computing and telecommunication industry, and so far this continues to be the state-of-affairs. This is appalling as computers are not very useful in the absence of good software applications to run on them. We are very far behind other countries (even Britain and Australia are much further along) in this important technology sector. Three-quarters of all British primary care physicians currently have a practice management computer system. This is even more depressing in light of the fact that Canada is becoming a leader in other software sectors (graphics, visualization, robotics).

Software manufacturing should be a very attractive investment sector compared to many industries, as it is relatively inexpensive on a cost-per-job-created basis. Software jobs have start-up costs that are only a fraction of manufacturing or service sector jobs. It is not too late but we must start immediately. Government is not going to have all the ideas needed to get this industry moving. Recently even Premier Bob Rae agreed that Ontario could do more to develop businesses based on environmental technologies and healthcare and in computer software, and this is in spite of his government putting a hold on some of the previous government's medical computing initiatives!

In Canada, most healthcare research and development funding has traditionally been directed to non-profit organizations, usually university associated researchers. While many creative people are associated with these environments, as many or more creative people work in the for-profit sector. More importantly, the market orientation of the for-profit sector tends to result in more practical products that are highly attentive to market need and user input. This preoccupation by government with the non-profit academic sector must change, or at least be balanced by equal sharing of projects with private enterprise. The province of Quebec seems to be far ahead at exploiting this opportunity.

Telecommunications

Although Canada is a world leader in this industry, the impact in the health sector has been minimal to date. A small and successful Telemedicine Canada project out of The Toronto Hospital is helping continuing medical education across the country. Currently it is delivering 900 programs per year mostly to hospitals. About 25% are directed to doctors (in hospitals), the rest to hospitals, nurses, and allied health professional audiences. Recently it has reached beyond Canada to the U.S. and some Carribbean audiences. Little has been done to try and develop systems for supporting rural healthcare beyond the aforementioned educational application.

Although satellites have now been used in test studies to allow medical experts to review CT and MRI and X-ray data from very remote locations, these telecommunication *tours-de-force* have not proven to be cost-effective. Such links have even allowed specialists in big city medical centres to examine patients half a world away, but, once again the current costs make such applications prohibitively expensive.

A National Health Information Utility and Network

We have demonstrated that the public's interest in medical information knows no limit. Each year the amount of new information doctors are expected to digest grows more and more unmanageable. Most physicians fell behind long ago. Today the task of keeping technically current is virtually impossible. No physician, specialist or generalist, knows all that he or she needs to know in his or her own area of interest, let alone what is happening in medical science generally. Everyone tries the best one can, but it is a losing proposition. In Canada, family physicians receive 10-20 different medical journals per month, many of which get a quick glance and then go into the circular file. Not much of what is in these journals is of major significance, mostly it's just good updating review articles by specialists or academics on timely topics of wide interest. But some of the material is very important. There is never enough time to read even this material. Specialists have a narrower domain to try and keep up with, and even then it is an impossible task.

Somehow, we all believe that eventually technology will have to provide a solution. Is this a realistic possibility? An unqualified yes! The various technological elements to implement this are currently available off-the-shelf. "Eventually" doesn't just happen, we have to plan it. What is missing is the national strategy and the will.

What purpose would such a system serve? It could act as a clearinghouse for what is currently medically possible and where to get it. It could provide a lot of information, saving millions of dollars in informational visits to doctors' offices. It could help minimize the wastage. It could serve to keep health professionals apprised of the current state of the art in every specialty of medicine, thus assuring quality or effective care. While knowing everything is a desirable expectation of their doctors by the public, it has never been, nor will it likely become a reality with the present system. **A health utility and network could bring knowing almost everything much closer to reality.**

What are some of the barriers to a National Health Information Utility? To use an information utility (even if the database/s were available) currently requires knowledge of computer and telecommunication protocols. Typically, one logs on to the system through a modem link to the telephone. The modem is increasingly built-in to computers available at consumer electronic retail outlets. This skill is gradually becoming a part of regular education. In the next year or so we can expect the user interface to become simplified and more widespread in use. Much effort is currently being directed towards simplifying the dial-up process.

Another important barrier on the health professional side is the time required by nurse or doctor or other provider to search or use the system. Unlike many non-medical professionals (lawyer, architect, engineer, accountant, journalist, corporate librarian), who are paid to do informational searching, there is no current provision in the fee schedule for physician case-preparation time, or documentation or information search time. Even if the best system imaginable existed, few doctors would use it unless it was cost-effective. If such a proposed system is to become a reality, this aspect of information utility use must be addressed.

Paranoia about confidentiality of medical information has definitely slowed the use of computers. This is a major hurdle. Fear of litigation is another problem. There is a well known adage amongst medical computing pioneers involved in artificial intelligence (AI), or knowledge-based computer applications, specifically stand-alone applications, that goes: 300,000 lawyers are waiting in the wings to sue the developer for the first little old lady who dies as a result of using some medical AI program in a drug store. This threat has been a major impediment to the rapid diffusion of such software.

More challenging than training in the use of the system is the creation of the Health Database/s. This would require the collaboration of a number of medical, pharmaceutical and computer experts in a critical mass of ongoing database builders and managers. Although earlier discussions in the book indicated the difficulty of hammering out consensus amongst medical professionals, it should be very much simpler to achieve this in Canada than in the U.S. The system can start small and grow over time. If this is the era of information workers, why isn't this sector a target for job-creation and investment? **I don't understand why the public isn't demanding the information systems needed to keep them up to date.**

Why has no such system materialized before now? Cost, national or provincial will, specific project vision, and large project management skills, have been in short supply. Until now there were technological limitations but most of these barriers are rapidly disappearing. There have been a few attempts at much smaller scale systems, all have failed, and most were commercial efforts directed only at doctors. None have had the scope proposed. The American Medical Association has sunk $25 million into physician telecommunication experiments over the past ten years without success.

Canada's Modern Medicine Online (MMOL):
A Brief, Unsuccessful Try

In Canada, Southam Communications tried a very simple bulletin board system (BBS), Modern Medicine OnLine (MMOL), for doctors one year ago without success. **It was offered free to any doctor** from British Columbia to Newfoundland, but after one year's pilot effort it was discontinued. Discussions with the manager of this venture (whose job was terminated with the demise of the service) indicated that telecommunication costs were too expensive, and system usage was never broad enough to attract hoped-for commercial sponsors.

Of the 1,400 doctors (total doctors in Canada 50,000) who registered as subscribers to MMOL, fewer than a hundred regulars used the system more than 10-20 times for any purpose. Most of them felt the medical information available on the system was modestly useful but not compelling. The most enjoyable aspect for most doctors was the ability to send messages back and forth to colleagues, and most users were struck with how well the system catalyzed communication amongst perfect strangers. **This aspect of breaking down the isolation of doctors across the country in their offices is terribly important.** I truly miss sitting down to MMOL each morning with my coffee and looking at my daily messages. Perhaps in retrospect, these early efforts simply occurred before the market was ready. All the right stakeholders were not brought in from conception, and finally the mix of services might not have been correct. This author has made an ongoing study of these types of initiatives, and intuition suggests the time is now very much more appropriate for another attempt, provided the correct elements are included.

Who are the stakeholders? The public, government, health professionals of many types (nurse, pharmacist, doctor, allied medical professionals), the pharmaceutical, telecommunication and computer industries. Governments will have to subsidize such a project, and ideally the directors would be a consortium of federal and provincial health ministry personnel together with an advisory committee of technical experts. This must be a national initiative, as it would be available across the country as a national health information asset. Perhaps the Science Council of Canada or the Canadian Institute for Advanced Research could act as catalysts? Perhaps a large computer software company partner could be found to joint venture? Much could be subcontracted to small firms.

To greatly simplify the dial-up process, patients and doctors might access the system by taking advantage of the new Health Card in use in Ontario and other provinces. Those provinces not currently using such a card might follow eventually. Alternatively a Visa or Mastercard might do. Any card with a magnetic strip could allow access with a simple sweep of the card through a cheap magnetic strip card reader. Eventually, the telephone alone might work when voice-response systems are perfected. Initially a computer interface will be necessary. Although only half of Canadian doctors have a computer in their office today, their number is growing rapidly. The public has many fewer computers and, although this is also changing, access for the patients will need some thought. Almost all Canadian hospitals and libraries have such equipment. For citizens not owning a computer, certain public locations could easily be identified for such access: place-of-employment, labs, hospitals, public health offices, doctors offices, and libraries.

What type of information might be available in this national health information utility? There would be many categories or modular databases constructed in phases. For doctors, one database might act as an electronic version of *Current Therapy*, a book (out-of-date by the time it is printed) that is revised annually and lists the current treatments for almost every known medical problem. Several such textbooks are available, and while not perfect therapy references, they are a starting point for the consensual current therapy reference database to be created by our Canadian health experts. With such a database, a physician could, very rapidly, interrogate the system for the latest treatment for AIDS, syphilis, tropical diseases, pneumonia, diabetes, high cholesterol, arthritis, prostate problems, whatever. Patients could similarly access the same information (or an abstracted version) and thus confirm that they were getting the latest and standard treatment, and thus possibly reduce the expense resulting from double-doctoring.

Optimal Drug Therapy Database

A recent report from the Science Council of Canada, *Medication and Health Policy: A Research Agenda*, calls for new ways for pharmaceuticals to be marketed, prescribed, dispensed, consumed and regulated because of the rising cost of healthcare. If healthcare providers and consumers are to achieve the goal of optimal drug therapy, which is defined as medication that is clinically appropriate and accessible to all who need it, and at a cost that society is willing to bear, we need:

- more effective collection, dissemination, and use of information on the benefits and risks of individual drugs;
- processes to assess the value of new drugs to the individual patient and to the healthcare system;
- integrated provincial health databases to be used as a foundation for population-based research on drug use;
- improved skills in educating health professionals about critical assessment and health outcome evaluation;
- recognition by the physician of the patient's right to participate in medical decisions;
- more education and information to realign consumer attitudes and expectations to reflect realistic goals for drug therapy.

This report confirms the need for the types of databases recommended in this chapter. The report also confirms that there seems almost no limit to the creative capacity of science and technology to develop new drug technologies. But, it says there are limits to what the healthcare system can afford and to what treatments Canadians are willing to accept. Here I disagree.

While there are definitely limits to what the government healthcare system as currently defined and configured can afford, **there are no limits to what people are prepared to go after when they believe it is essential or even desirable,** in or out of the defined health system boundaries. It is impossible to try and limit this behaviour, other than by the constraint of individual ability to pay.

A drug treatment cost-comparison database, that would be of great interest to consumers, might include choices in drug treatment in which cost of therapy was indicated. Included in such a comparison could be the comparative efficacy of a selected range of drugs from the newest to the oldest for each condition (common problems for which multiple options were available). Thus those paying for their drugs would be able to decide on the basis of cost-effectiveness. Doctors know that for most illnesses, many drugs might be selected. It would be very useful if a person not able to afford a more recent drug could be reassured that several other less expensive products have essentially the same effectiveness.

A database that contains comparative pricing, in addition to having reference treatment information, could also provide background on all diseases, and thus patients could learn more about their particular illness. A special section on emerging health technologies could keep patients with medical problems, for which a definitive treatment is not yet available, aware of advances. Such a system could disseminate new discoveries almost instantaneously. It could act as a reference against which people could check some of the wild claims appearing in popular media. **A national health information utility would be a true national treasure.**

Other Services the Health Information Utility Might Provide

An important part of the treatment section of the health information utility for each disease would be statistics on success rates of competing techniques, if one method is not definitive. Comparative data from hospital to hospital might also be made available, injecting elements of competition.[1] A good example is the study of the relative outcomes of alternative cataract procedures reported in *Ophthalmology*, June 1991. Analysis of over 600,000 cataract extractions in the U.S. found that patients who underwent ICCE (intracapsular cataract extraction and phacoemulsification) were 1.5 times as likely to be rehospitalized because of retinal detachment within four years of surgery than ECCE patients (extracapsular cataract extraction). In Canada presently, ECCE is more common than ICCE as the equipment for ICCE is more expensive. Is the saving in the cost of equipment purchased exceeded by the cost of the extra hospitalization?

Resident within this database would be useful guides to regular wellness topics. Diet in normal and abnormal situations, exercise advice for every age and for those with specific health problems. Information about equipment for recreational exercise and assistive devices for the disabled could equally easily be part of such a system. Canadian libraries could conceivably list the health titles available in their collections.

Of particular usefulness in such a database would be known risk factors associated with those diseases for which such data exists. Information pertaining to modifiable risk factors could assist the public and doctors to minimize whatever risks are subject to such voluntary control. This is a huge area of opportunity.

Comparisons of hospitals regarding infection rates, typical success rates for various surgical procedures, etc. could serve to stimulate competition and excellence and thus further quality assurance.

Small portions of this kind of information are actually available in the U.S., available only to subscribers at a fee, in a number of diverse commercial systems such as: Dialog, Compuserve, and Prodigy, but not in anywhere near the coherent and usable format envisioned here.

Should the Canadian system be free or should there be a charge? This is a very interesting and contentious issue and would require considerable thought. There probably must be a charge. It would have to be low enough to encourage use, compared to sources of free information elsewhere, and yet high enough to help to pay for the system's continued development. The quality of the information in the system would be greater than free material. Incentives would have to be put in place to create interest in system usage. A good possibility would be that legal requirements would evolve mandating the regular use of such systems at each medical encounter.

There would be many markets for such an information utility beyond the health system. It would represent a resource for the educational system. Business users would be target markets. Again, methods of payment might be similar to other well-known existing information utilities such as Dialog.

I discussed earlier in this book (Chapter 4) the growing importance of medical management guidelines. Some commentators, in fact, have labelled the 1990s as the era of guideline development. A guideline database would be a natural application for the systems discussed in this chapter.

In the U.S., until recently, guideline development was haphazard and poorly coordinated. In 1989 Congress established the Agency for Health Care Policy and Research (AHCPR) to improve the quality, appropriateness and effectiveness of healthcare. AHCPR has taken over responsibility for guideline development originally started by the National Institute of Health's Consensus Development Program.

When and how is Canada going to address this challenge? As I have mentioned, we will either accept the American guidelines, if we can afford to implement them, or we develop our own less expensive guidelines, and widen the *guideline gap*. Example: in the U.S. currently, any insured athlete, amateur or professional, who injures a knee sufficiently to require continuing medical attention, will receive an MRI (magnetic resonance imaging) screening procedure before arthroscopy (examination of the inside of the joint under anaesthesia by arthroscope) would be contemplated. In the U.S. it is malpractice to do arthroscopy first. In Canada, with very limited access to MRI, arthroscopy is the initial procedure of choice.

Medical Mind-Net: A First Step

The MMOL experience has one interesting and potentially useful lesson. MMOL catalyzed physician collegiality and inter-communication. MMOL reduced physician isolation. MMOL allowed diverse types of medical personnel to help each other in ways not previously experienced. Telephones don't do this, Faxes don't do this, letter writing is too slow. There is something entirely new that electronic mail makes possible, and this is the creation of a mind-net.

When I was monitoring the progress of MMOL, I would occasionally throw out requests for help on different subjects, some medical, some having to do with how physicians used their computers. Always, to a varying degree, there would be rapid responses and then, like ripples from a pebble tossed into a lake, the response activity would flourish for a brief time and disappear. The ability to tap the vast experiential resource that Canadian physicians as a group represent is mind-boggling to contemplate. This could be in effect a collective database of the best medical minds in Canada. Harnessing such a resource, while a huge undertaking, could have amazing potential.

Compact Disc Databases (CD-ROM): Possible Staging Tools

While the creation of a national network as described is a very large undertaking, smaller aspects of this project could be immediately created and implemented and distributed on compact discs (CD-ROM). This technology is just starting to gain momentum after more than a decade of development. A single CD-ROM (looks the same as the music disks but contains text instead) can contain up to 250,000 full pages of text; such disks are now becoming a popular distribution medium for many large databases. For example, the U.S. National Library of Medicine's *Index Medicus* is available on CD-ROM and can be used on any desktop computer equipped with a CD-ROM reader. Such readers are available now for less than $500. These devices are similar to musical compact disc players, but they are specially designed to read digital data rather than play music. Incidentally, some add the capacity to play music, as well as the data function, since the electronics are identical to the music device but with better error detection.

The only problem with fixed media such as CD-ROM is that once the data is placed on such a disk it is unchanging, and thus regular updates or a subscription to provide continuing up-to-date information are necessary. Single discs can be reproduced for only a few dollars, a fraction of the cost of the identical data on paper. There is tremendous potential for CD-ROM technology in medicine, law, and science.

Interactive Videos:
Patients in the Treatment Decision Making Process

At The Toronto Hospital, a group of patients with Benign Prostatic Hypertrophy (BPH), in layman's language an enlarged prostate, have been involved in a recent study in which they make the treatment choice once they learn their options. The BPH interactive video, *Choosing: Prostatectomy or Watchful Waiting,* provides outcome probabilities for prostate surgery versus watchful waiting, using specific information on the patient. Linked to the videodisc machine, the computer is programmed with the latest data on the disease and the outcomes of each treatment option, generating 250 possible patient scenarios.

The patient is given a printout of the risk/benefit analysis for his specific situation for each choice. Of the 26 patients in the Toronto program in May, 1991, none chose surgery afterward. Patients seem to be more risk averse than surgeons. The program has since been on hold awaiting the opening of the new Prostate Centre at the hospital. The cost of developing such educational tools is high, but they may well pay for themselves and should be marketable internationally.

The prostate video is the first in a series from the nonprofit Foundation For Informed Medical Decision Making in Hanover, New Hampshire. A team from the University of Toronto Health Administration Department is working on the design for a cardiovascular disease video, with support from both the foundation and the Ontario Ministry of Health. Obviously the desire is to reduce cardiovascular surgery for people with stable angina (known pain due to coronary artery narrowing, but currently stable). Costing $7 million per program, this seems a very pricey way to dissuade patients but may be cost-effective in the long run.

According to Joseph Kasper, the CEO of the Foundation for Informed Medical Decision Making, they hope to produce 25 to 30 programs in the next few years. A program for back problems is due in the fall of 1992 and a breast program soon after.

In the U.S., Blue Cross is so intrigued with the prostate program that they will be trying a test which pays doctors $50 for each showing in lieu of a costlier second opinion. Currently a hardware configuration set up for viewing these special videos costs a doctor/clinic about $8,000 (US). While this type of informed decision assistance is an excellent idea whose time is coming, unless doctors can charge for such informational encounters I don't know many Canadian doctors who would be prepared to spend this much money for an educational tool. The earlier patient education video tapes were a major flop economically for the original entrepreneurs. I also hope the Canadians who are participating in the cardiovascular disease video disk will receive a decent royalty for their involvement if and when such programs receive wide distribution and usage.

CHAPTER 14

THE NEW ECONOMY: DOES CANADA WANT TO PARTICIPATE?

In *The Third Wave*, Alvin Toffler describes how the new world economic order is being driven by information technologies, and how the computer and biotech sectors, together with telecommunications, are two of the fastest growing sectors in most countries.[1] The potential for capitalizing on these factors seems to have been completely lost on Canadians and Canadian health officials. While American, European, Far Eastern and other innovators have been creating huge enterprises based on health technology applications, Canadian officials have chosen to simply import these technologies. Thus, Canada has a very minimal local health high technology sector. The excuse has always been we are too small and we can't compete. Meanwhile, Israel, with a population of less than 4 million, has developed contenders in some of the world's leading health technologies. Elscint, the premier Israeli imaging company, competes successfully with General Electric, Phillips and Siemens for a part of the lucrative and rapidly-growing imaging market. Competing is a matter of political will, not technical competence. Canada has some of the best scientific minds available, but many are leaving for the U.S.

Whether we like it or not, medicine is going to be technologically-driven for the indefinite future. Information-intensive fields like medicine will by definition be technology-intensive. Too many international economists and technology planners have recognized the trend to The New Economy in computers, telecommunications, medicine and biotechology for us to ignore it. If we don't have the forecasting powers to anticipate the health products and services that science will create in the next ten years, let alone twenty, and the role of the health and technology sector of the future, how are we to plan to pay for them? The creation of Canadian national wealth by innovation and enterprise in healthcare and other sectors is the only hope.

Advances do not come from wishful thinking, from alternative healers or gurus in sandals. Wisdom perhaps, but not a cure for cancer or AIDS, or the development of gene defect or gene mutation repair. Scientific medicine and healing must coexist. Caring and compassion and scientifically-based, efficacious medicine are not mutually exclusive. However, if the Canadian public wants a different vision of healthcare, a low-tech Third World vision, so be it. It will certainly cost a lot less, but it will not contribute much to the survival of our economy.

Biotechnology

In *BusinessWeek*, March 2, 1992, the cover says it all, "Biotech: America's Dream Machine." This industry is predicted to generate a $50 billion economy alone worldwide by the early 2000s. For ten years only a risky and expensive gamble, the pay-off is now arriving. Currently it is estimated that biotech companies have some 100 drugs in human trials and more than 400 products in some stage of development.

Biotech companies are involved in manipulating the very processes of life at the cellular and subcellular genetic material levels. The products pouring from this crucible are novel compared to older pharmaceutical methods. Whereas drugs are rather "global" in their effects on human physiological processes, the newer biotech products are very much more specific in their effects. The trend is to therapeutic effects targetted at much smaller physiological domains of human biological functioning.

The industry is driven by rapid advances in the identification of human, animal, and plant genes. Of the 50,000 to 100,000 predicted human genes, fewer than 2 percent have been isolated. Immunology is advancing rapidly with the huge amounts of R & D carried out to find a cure for AIDS over the past eight years. Companies with "immune" in their name (Immunex, ImmuLogic, ImmunoGen, Immunomedics, MedImmune, Immune Response) are only a few of the new companies in the disease-fighting arena.

It is impossible to keep all the names and products straight. I will review briefly some current product categories and company names to give you a sampling of the starting line-up.

Gene-Splicing to Create Proteins Normally Produced in Humans

We have already discussed EPO or erythropoietin, which stimulates marrow to produce more red cells, and G-CSF or granulocyte stimulating factor. Alpha Interferon is used for healing herpes and hepatitis and is being tried out on AIDS. Others break up blood clots, speed wound healing and fight infections. These are products of recombinant DNA technology which employs gene-splicing technologies to produce discrete proteins that perform critical processes in the body. Just a few of the companies doing recombinant DNA research are: Amgen, Amylin, Biogen, Calbio, Chiron, Genentech, Genetics Institute, Gensia, Genzyme, Imclone, Immunex, Regeneron, Repligen, Synergen, T Cell Sciences, Xoma.

Biotech Vaccines (Recombinant DNA Technology)

Chiron, Genlabs, Immune Response, MedImmune, Repligen, North American Vaccine.

Carbohydrate Chemistry

Some sugar molecules in the body signal to cells and the immune system, which helps in fighting and suppressing inflammatory reactions. Sometimes the body over-reacts and produces too much causing diseases like rheumatoid arthritis. New drugs will help modulate all this. Companies in this area include: Alpha-beta, Biogen, Cytel, Genentech, Genzyme, Glycomed, Icos.

In Canada, Hyal Pharmaceutical is just starting to explore the role of hyaluronic acid, a so-called proteoglycans molecule which seems to be very useful as a carrier in transporting other medications bound to it to areas of inflammation (joints, muscles, etc.).

Antisense Molecules:
Chemicals that Selectively Block Messages in DNA

Errant messages inside the body can cause disease. The strategy, thus, is to sabotage disease-causing genes by sending in chemicals, modeled after DNA, that act as chemical switches and stop these genes from working. Such antisense molecules could prevent AIDS viruses from replicating in the body and short-circuit disorders such as Huntington's disease and sickle-cell anaemia. Companies pursuing this approach: Gilead, Isis, Genta, Triplex, Hybridon.

New methods of "rational drug design" can shorten the older random screening of chemicals for potential drugs to identify the most appropriate candidates for drugs. The new area of receptor chemistry has vast potential for new treatments. Soluble receptors, or the actual isolated part of a cell that is normally the site of attachment for a specific chemical, can be genetically produced independent of the rest of the cell wall! Theoretically, such proteins can be used per se therapeutically! Expect progress in this area from: Agouron, Alkermes, Athena, Cambridge Neuroscience, Cephalon, Genelabs, Genentech, Neurogen, Oncogene Science, Vertex.

Antibodies

Antibodies are natural disease fighters when infections threaten the body. Viral infections, traditionally very tough to treat, may give way to advances in this area. Additionally, autoimmune illnesses are diseases such as thyroid disease, arthritis, multiple sclerosis, and lupus, where the immune system somehow identifies its own proteins as being foreign and starts to kill its own tissues by mistake. Products in this market can be expected from: Alkermes, Centocor, Chiron, Cor, Cytogen, Genelabs, Genentech, Idec, Imclone, ImmunoGen, Immunomedics, Repligen, T Cell Sciences, Tanox, Univax, Xoma.

Peptide Chemistry

Peptides are smaller and more stable molecules than the larger protein drugs that break down rapidly in the body. They have antibacterial properties and may have a role in infection treatments. R & D is underway in peptide chemistry at: Affymax, Centocor, Chiron, Cor Therapeutics, Icos, ImmuLogic, Magainin.

Cell Transplant/Gene Therapy

Finally, the most far-out approach to genetic disorders is to attempt to insert corrective genes into a part of the body that has some defective cells which are not making an essential substance: so-called cell transplant or gene therapy. The strategy is to transplant into the body either healthy or genetically altered cells to cure problems such as cancer, diabetes, AIDS, cystic fibrosis and a host of other gene-defect illnesses. The challenge in all this is how to get the correction to the right place. Although gene therapy is proceeding far more rapidly than most anticipated, much work needs to be done in this very complex area: Advanced Tissue Sciences, Applied Immune Sciences, Cellpro, Genetic Therapy, Somatix, Systemix, Viagene, Vical.

Selfcare Using Intelligent Monitoring Devices

Selfcare for diabetics started years ago with patients monitoring their urine with dipsticks for levels of urinary sugar. Prior to dipstick testing, dietary management and office-taken blood tests were the only monitoring and control methods. Doctor and patient used this very indirect data to plan diabetic control with insulin or oral medications. Ten years ago the earliest glucometers became available at high prices, allowing self-testing of blood sugar directly, using a finger-prick and several drops of blood. This simple development considerably improved diabetic treatment, monitoring, and planning. Today for less than $100 a diabetic can purchase a pen-sized glucometer to accomplish the same task. Other more sophisticated devices are available for Type I (insulin-dependent diabetes) that can actually compute and plan insulin injection doses and scheduling of injections based on a number of patient parameters. These devices have become more accurate and smarter (as microprocessors have been embedded inside to add logic), smaller, and less expensive. We are just beginning the era of patient self-monitoring.

Futrex, a company in Rockville, Maryland, recently announced a bloodless glucose monitoring device that does not require a drop of blood like the previous technologies.[2] It works on an optical sensing principle. The user simply puts a finger tip into the device and the sensor reads near infra-red light absorption through your skin to capillaries in the subcutaneous layer and indicates a glucose reading. The current test device needs considerable miniaturization to become a consumer product. Whether it will be as good or as inexpensive as existing reliable devices is too early to say. But self-test optical sensing may become a very big business.

We are all aware of electronic blood-pressure measuring devices, pulse-rate devices, and a host of new exercise-related self-use monitors (calories expended, etc.) flooding the market. Soon, blood sugar sensors will be joined by cholesterol testers and patient self-testers for a variety of other blood chemistry parameters. It is impossible to predict what will come next. To date the world of fitness and exercise devices seems to have most advanced the concept of self-monitoring.

What we can count on is that ALL these devices will get smarter and cheaper, at a pace we can barely imagine. Entire industries will be formed around these products. Some strategy for integrating them into the regular healthcare system will have to be found that best serves both the individual and the health professional, since patients currently have to get prescriptions from doctors for controlled drugs, and thus cannot yet be completely self-managing.

Enabling Technologies Impacting Medical Research and Healthcare

In the next few years, entirely new medical treatments will become available as a result of advances in the following key enabling technologies: supercomputers, massively parallel computers; powerful and less expensive workstation visualization tools; simulation; lasers; nanotechnology; genetic engineering.

Using the computational power of supercomputer and parallel machines, and extraordinary new Rational Drug Design software, entire new classes of drugs that are far better and safer than previous pharmaceutical products will start to swamp the sluggish and outdated bureaucracies of the U.S. Food and Drug Administration (FDA), and Canada's Health Protection Branch (HPB). Already bogged down and falling further and further behind in processing existing new drug applications, these organizations threaten to stall and delay truly advanced pharmaceutical products that can make life better for patients with lethal conditions as well as chronic disease sufferers.

Powerful workstations and emerging visualization software will enable doctors to plan and simulate operations and many other types of treatments and interventions before they are actually performed. As well, they will be able to explain in graphic detail to patients just exactly what might be done. Fifteen months from now, most of the complex 3-dimensional human anatomical databases necessary to support some of these systems will have been completed and such computer-based simulation tools will become available for doctors' offices and hospitals.[3] Simulation will become one of the largest applications of powerful workstation computers in healthcare.

Imaging: A Major Trend in Future Health Practices

No area in Canada has been more constrained in its growth than what is perhaps the most important innovation in medicine since the invention of the X-ray. Misperception by Canadian health planners of the potential enabling role of this technology is holding back Canada's healthcare industry. Modern medical imaging (Computed Tomography or CT, Magnetic Resonance Imaging or MRI, and Ultrasonic Imaging or UI) are in fact the most successful sophisticated applications of computers in medicine to date. People don't think of this as the computers are hidden to the user (built into the equipment). The market is dominated by American, European, and Japanese companies. This powerful technology has a much larger future than its current use in medical diagnosis alone, and Canada cannot afford to abandon this field to others.

Canada, in its continuing efforts to control costs, has in fact denied reasonable access by its citizens to this technology. In the U.S. recent estimates of the number of MRI installations are about 2,500. While this is probably too many, Canada's 25 MRI facilities are far too few according to many critics. Several British imaging experts believe the greatest future potential for imaging, particularly MRI, lies in its use in health screening programs, particularly cardiovascular screening.

We have touched the subject of screening earlier in Chapter 10. CT and particularly MRI are powerful non-invasive tools for potential application in the routine or periodic patient checkup. No pain, no danger, no messy hospital stay, with the potential for TOTAL BODY SCANNING on a regular basis. If that sounds too expensive, and it currently is, then focus just on a smaller imaging target, for example, the heart alone. Techniques for the fast MRI scanning of not only heart anatomy, but the functional aspects of heart muscle motion and its coronary artery status are rapidly evolving. In other words, we are not far from a method of non-invasive coronary artery examination in full 3-D! No dangerous coronary artery angiograms complete with arterial punctures by scary big needles, infusion of radiopacque dyes to allow the outlines of these vessels to be seen on X-rays, etc. Such MRI screens would be done periodically, and a computer would compare each subsequent set of images with previous ones. And this is only the beginning. Are we doomed to buying all this technology and related software from the U.S., Europe or Japan? I desperately hope not!

If the government will not let its medical scientists get on with developing the potential of this technology within Medicare, then it should help private enterprise to do it, or at least, not block private enterprise. We have barely scratched the surface in the types of applications that will flow from such technologies. Imaging and visualization are the future of a large part of medical practice. The potential of three-dimensional large-scale reconstructive rendering of data from CT, MRI and ultrasound are phenomenal. In fact, despite the odds, Canada currently has a leader in a piece of this market, ISG Technologies of Toronto.

ISG has recognized that machines like CT and MRI scanners, powerful and expensive as they are for medical imaging, are simply transducers. A transducer is a device that senses data and then either displays it or sends it to a computer for processing and display. The only difference between a thermometer or weight scale and an MRI is cost and **the amount of data it detects!** ISG develops and manufactures systems that use large amounts of digital imaging data from CT and MRI to allow doctors to diagnose, plan, and monitor treatment away from the actual CT or MRI machines on special ISG visualization workstations. Very recently, ISG workstations and *The Viewing Wand* ™ are being used during neurosurgical operations in the OR (operating room). This special probe allows much better localization of anatomical objects than previously possible. The amount of data an MRI can send to an ISG workstation is becoming astronomical in scope. A single one millimetre slice of your body represented in an MRI contains about one million bytes (a megabyte) of data. That is one millimetre. Multiply that by 64 (one 3-D data set) slices and you begin to get the scale of data assembly and manipulation going on in one of these three-dimensional imaging workstations! The great majority of ISG's sales are in the U.S, not in Canada. One wonders how long this company will stay resident in Canada?

The limited number of imaging facilities in Canada has restricted the potential of this technology for many other areas; veterinary medicine is just one. The potential of this technology combined with visualization workstations in education, sports, and other non-medical areas is limitless. It is anticipated that MRI systems, currently costing well over $1 million, will be superseded within 2-3 years by smaller systems that cost one-third to one-fifth of today's prices. These less expensive systems will be designed to be used on smaller anatomical targets, such as extremities (arm, leg), even finger joints, to monitor joint cartilage response to new arthritis medications non-invasively. These second generation MRI systems will be faster and thus allow many more patients to be processed in the same daily schedule. The widespread use of visualization workstations will evolve as doctors begin to use these powerful tools routinely. Imaging is one of the most important future fields for job creation if we would only wake up to the opportunity.

Recently breast MRI with special Gadolium-DTPA contrast has allowed fat tissue suppression resulting in much improved breast imaging which may change the way breast cancer is treated. This technique is currently expensive, but the price will come down with volume. It is expected that significant reductions in the number of expensive and distressing breast biopsies will result from this technique.

I was informed by a Toronto radiologist, during a recent interview, that his large radiology group had been unsuccessful in trying to set up a private imaging centre (CT, MRI, X-ray, etc.). The government had blocked their attempts to obtain a licence for their facility for any imaging services other than X-ray and ultrasound.

More unsettling still, than their failed attempt at a non-hospital imaging centre, was a story related to me by the same physician about a different group's unsuccessful attempt to set up a Sports Medicine Imaging Centre that would have offered Canadian (and American) athletes all the latest imaging technology **completely outside the Medicare system so it would not be a burden to government!**

Laser Scanning, Photodynamic Therapy, Confocal Microscopy

Until recently medical lasers have been used primarily to cut, burn, kill, disintegrate and vaporize various human tissues from skin to corneas (the transparent part of your eye) to kidney stones. As researchers are discovering ever more sophisticated means for controlling laser energy (pulse width, frequency, etc.), the number of applications besides simple tissue destruction have been growing rapidly.

Some very clever physicists in the U.S. have even proposed a means to screen for superficial and deep breast masses as small as one millimetre using unimaginably short femtosecond laser pulse bursts in a complex imaging system.[4] (A microsecond is one-millionth of a second, a picosecond is a billionth, a femtosecond, a trillionth of a second!) Since breast cancer is continuing to rise (15,500 cases diagnosed in Canada in 1990, and 5,000 deaths) in our population, and continues to defy medical science's attempts to come up with better treatment, early detection looks like the best approach. Mammography has limitations. It is hoped these new tools might improve our diagnostic capabilities in this very difficult area.

Very recently lasers have been used to treat certain kinds of cancers utilizing Photodynamic Therapy (PDT). In this type of treatment, relatively low powered laser pulses (compared to the previously mentioned higher energy level vaporizing bursts) are delivered to lesions inside bladder, bowel, or deep into thicker tissues with fibre-optic guides. The patient has first been treated with a drug called Photofrin II developed by British Columbia's Quadra Logic Technologies Inc. (at the moment a leader in this field). Photofrin is a photosensitizer of certain tissues, particularly cancerous tissues. When the tissue is subject to intense laser light, cancer-killing toxins called singlet-oxygen are created by the photoactive chemicals in the tissue and delivered preferentially to the cancerous tissue, sparing normal tissues which do not take up this photosensitizer in as concentrated amounts. Thus the cancers are destroyed with very little side effect. Expect to see many developments in this area.

Lasers can be used not only for zapping tissues, but for measurement and control. We have not begun to exploit their potential in scanning body surfaces, creating 3-D computer models that can be used for simulation. To date most of these applications have been in industrial processes. Their role in studying human motion is just beginning.

Confocal microscopy is an exciting new application area using lasers built-in to laboratory microscopes and enabling researchers to use visualization workstations (such as ISG's) in entirely new ways to reconstruct the cellular and subcellular world and study this magnified microscopic world in 3-D.

Molecular Nanotechnology: Molecular Manufacturing

This is a very new area of science dedicated to the creation of devices that are constructed from the manipulation of matter at the molecular level – molecular engineering. The goal is to replace existing industries, with their huge plants and processes that manipulate matter from the top down, with small, pollution-free facilities that manufacture devices from the molecular level or from the bottom up. A controversial scientist, Eric Drexler, has been a leading force in this field, and recently wrote a book, *Unbounding the Future: The Nanotechnology Revolution.* Although the potential for this field may take decades to be realized, some of the tools are now in place for rapid advances in medicine. The journal *Science* devoted almost one-half of its November 29, 1991 issue to this subject.

Probably the first area of major impact of nanotechnology in medicine will be the biosensor field, a merging of modern physical chemistry, optics, microelectronics, biotechnology and computers to provide Star Trek-like medical tools.

Biosensors

The most common application of sensors in medicine to date have been pressure-sensors that can be used during operations or in intensive care units to sense intra-arterial blood pressure. These devices have been getting smaller and cheaper over time. Lucas Novasensor, a California firm, makes a blood-pressure sensor that is little bigger than a grain of salt. Now other tiny and smart sensor devices are emerging which combine laser optics and biochemistry to detect not only a growing number of blood chemistry elements such as glucose (sugar), electrolytes (sodium, potassium, chloride), liver and muscle enzymes, cholesterol, triglycerides, HDL-cholesterol, and uric acid. But more amazingly, such sensors can detect antigen-antibody reactions which occur when foreign bacterial and other agents invade our blood and interact with our immune systems!

It is hoped that in the future, these current invasive sensors, which must be passed through a needle into the blood, can be replaced in some cases by optical or other modalities which are non-invasive. It is a tremendous challenge, but the payoff will be immense.

Clinical Trials: The Engines of Pharmaceutical Change

It has already been noted that the pharmaceutical industry is generating new drug products faster than they can be approved and adopted. While many drugs causing the backlogs at Canada's Health Protection Branch are simply **me too** products that copy current drugs, a growing number are far superior to existing drugs and many are brand new with no existing analogues.

The world-wide annual clinical trial business is currently a $146 billion a year industry! Clinical trials are central to the process of getting a drug to the marketplace after it has been demonstrated to be effective and safe in the laboratory. It can cost a pharmaceutical company more than $100 million to bring a new drug from first concept to market. This is partly due to exhaustive toxicology and screening procedures to ensure safety, but increasingly it is due to the public's attitude of zero tolerance for risk or side effects and the growing cost of clinical trials delays all of this.

Canada, with its highly organized and efficient health system, is not getting a big enough share of this growing global clinical trial industry. Canada's current piece of this profitable and job-creating industry is a respectable $4 billion, but this is not enough and we could easily handle double or triple the amount of work if we recognized this as a national goal. Even more unacceptable is that much of the current clinical trial business done in Canada is handled by American or other foreign-owned subsidiaries. A major barrier to achieving a larger piece of this market is the problem of specialist saturation. This happens when the number of clinical trials exceeds the capacity of specialist participants to handle the new load. Partly this is due to limited numbers of a certain type of specialist, and partly to the distribution and organization of specialists at certain centres. Bringing more of this business to Canada might make smaller centres more attractive to specialists.

CHAPTER 15

WHY HEALTHCARE SHOULD BE THE BIGGEST INDUSTRY ON EARTH

We Cannot Afford a Healthcare Monopoly in the Fourth Wave

As the full impact of the shifting health paradigm sinks in around the world, governments are increasingly recognizing that national economic survival will depend on a degree of, but not total, withdrawal from monopolistic national health systems.

According to some, the ideal system of healthcare would be one paid for from general tax revenue which provided the individual with access to unlimited amounts of effective care. Many Canadians would like to put their collective heads in the sand and continue as is, hoping that the medical advances of the future that will enhance and prolong their lives will be available at current or lower cost to the nation. We want miraculous new transfers of Federal funds to sustain the provincial treasuries. In spite of warnings for years that the public and the health professionals were going to have to limit demands on the system to avoid our current crisis, no one altered his or her behavior. We all personally know of cases of abuse, but we tend to condone or ignore them.

And now, even if Canada were to direct the entire national treasury towards the funding of the health system, there still would not be enough money to pay for on-demand health service to all with no personal fiscal responsibility. This view does not even take into consideration the growing tax revolt, the shrinking tax base or the eroding economy that are present realities of life in Canada.

According to Marx, capitalism, with its singular power to galvanize human greed, inventiveness and innovation, would make possible the wide availability of products at an affordable price which socialism could then distribute more equitably. National healthcare systems currently find themselves caught somewhere in the middle. While science in capitalist societies continues to make a plethora of technical riches available to healthcare professionals and consumers, the industrial revolution that gave the world affordable automobiles and desktop computers has not been duplicated in the delivery of health services or products. The health system struggles to keep up with biologists and engineers in its attempt to absorb new technologies but it cannot decide whether the potential of each new offering to deliver improved levels of quality healthcare is real or imaginary. Meanwhile, no one has figured out a way to turn off the technological bubble machine.

Only the modern pharmaceutical industry has been able to achieve economies of scale in delivering new and useful medications to the millions at bearable prices and even that is far from universally the case. Drugs are only part of the healthcare system, albeit an increasingly expensive part (14.1% of all health dollars in 1990). The reasons why new drugs cost so much are complex and debatable. While drugs that might be used by millions are subject to market forces and get cheaper (aspirin, antibiotics), many drugs are only used by very small populations of patients (growth factor for leukemia, erythropoietin for chronic renal conditions, etc.). Because some of these are produced by biological rather than chemical processes, their prices remain higher, unless many other uses can be found which then result in economies of scale.

While MacDonalds figured out how to deliver relatively good quality food to the millions cost-effectively, we do not have an analogue in healthcare delivery. Healthcare is a labour-intensive activity which has resisted every attempt to make it more like other industries. While hamburgers, cars and computers are all products of various complexity, health services are the most complex mixture of human activities and technologies ever assembled by mankind. What adds an even greater level of complexity is medical science's incredible dependency on new information and knowledge. This is now exploding at an exponential rate. The medical knowledge base is currently doubling every two to five years. We are still very far away from an industrial or even post-industrial paradigm within which healthcare might be delivered or made available with any economies of scale. Worst of all, most countries (Canada included) view healthcare as a sector that consumes national wealth rather than as something that both consumes and creates wealth.

The futurist, Alvin Toffler, in his bestseller *The Third Wave*, described the post-industrial or Information Society (ours) as the result of a third wave of human evolution. The first was the agricultural revolution, while the second was the industrial revolution. The most important forces in what I will call the Fourth Wave of social evolution will be preoccupation with health, wellness and preventive measures, optimizing life extension, protection of the environment, information and molecular biology (unravelling of the genetic code). Where will Canada be in the Fourth Wave?

What We Really Need:
Restructuring, Innovation, Market Forces

All agree that health is more than the availability of healthcare services and is a desirable human state which is the final result of clean and prosperous economic environments, employment (preferably fulfilling), healthy family and other relationships and healthy lifestyles. However, in spite of the awareness of all these important factors, people still have bad genes, become ill, experience abuse, addictions, suffer emotional and mental illness, get injured, die prematurely from a host of causes and die for certain in the fullness of time. Many government health policy analysts maintain that our system can provide ALL necessary and effective medical interventions. As we have seen, this is not likely since the number of such services is rapidly increasing. Whether we call it Medicare, Healthcare, Catastrophic Care, Wellness Care, Holistic Health, Preventive Health or whatever, it will be too large a universe to be contained any longer within the domain of a single government funder. We must, therefore, redefine and delineate what healthcare services and products government will provide and what the private sector will supply.

Our federal government has begun to limit jurisdictionally what the healthcare budget will be. This begins the introduction into the healthcare equation of market forces and, hopefully, of alternative sources of funding. We cannot continue to allow a narrowly conceived philosophy of care to limit the horizons of our health system in the future. What we are absolutely NOT going to get from a pared down health system, with doctors on salary and many in CHC/HSO's, is better service. If you want to see the long-term ramifications of this approach look at the healthcare systems in the now defunct USSR and eastern Europe. Health professionals must not be excluded from entrepreneuring if we are to have alternatives, responsiveness and innovation.

A Mixture of Public and Private Services

From now on and into the future, a more realistic approach includes reduction of health system waste where possible, conservation of limited health resources, preventive measures that are known to reduce costs and/or improve the quality of life, protection against catastrophic illness, and multiple options for accessing as many additional services and products as one wants. This should be a mix of government and private enterprise to encourage competition and innovation. Most importantly, it should act as a stimulus to balance consumption of national wealth in healthcare by the creation of national wealth in new health related and other industries.

The U.S. health system, with all its shortcomings, is still the indisputable medical innovator on the globe. Rigid, monopolistic, centralized health bureaucracies have not been able to innovate or adapt. Even Monique Begin, Minister of National Health and Welfare, 1977-1984, and tireless crusader for Medicare in Canada, admitted that our system is rigid and resistant to innovation and change. Canada's system excludes competition, rejects profit motives entirely and rewards mediocrity. As well, with no competition, there is no second source or supplier when the monopoly starts to fail. Health monopolies are static structures, and like their political counterparts, are coming apart around the globe. Monopolies do not need to innovate, compete, reform or adapt. Also, as in Russia and eastern Europe, turning an entrenched state medical system into one that is market driven, will be difficult.

Before Bell Canada was deregulated, the price of a telephone was over $100. Now you can get a free telephone with a magazine subscription! This is not to suggest the analogy is that simple in healthcare, but we must try to inject more market forces into the medical system.

In the current Medicare system, there is only one source of payment for health services – the government. This principle is enforced by legislation and excludes any extra-billing. Few Canadians are even aware of the fact that, for example, in Ontario there is an act governing the licencing of imaging facilities. If an entrepreneur had an idea for setting-up a private imaging facility, and had the private financing, the law prohibits such a venture. It is all right for a Canadian on a long waiting list to pay $1,300 (of his/her own money) for an MRI scan in Buffalo. He or she can't spend the money in Toronto.

In 1984, the Canada Health Act, and subsequent provincial legislation prohibiting extra-billing, made it illegal for doctors to charge extra for any benefit of the plan. However, those healthcare services not a benefit can be paid for privately. Thus, for example, cosmetic surgery is a private item. Although there are few services not currently part of the plan, there is some variation from province to province about what is covered and what is not. The simplest way to privatize services more and more has been to delist selected Medicare benefits, which then would become the domain of private health payments.

Most governments (particularly Canada's) have avoided trying to come up with a list of insured essential services (while arbitrarily and secretly limiting them). As we have noted, the American state of Oregon has had the courage to define a basic health package with considerable input from citizens and health professionals. Health services or procedures outside this core package will be options, depending on government's ability to pay. The concept depends on a continual re-evaluation by an independent body of what the plan delivers as a function of local and national economic circumstances. The conceptual barrier has now been overcome and other governments can talk openly about the idea with some comfort.

There has been a lot of controversy about the Oregon Plan and it will continue. However, what is important is the pioneering efforts by one government to come to grips with the universal problem of government health benefits and exclusions in a world where financial limits exist. As the current belt-tightening becomes more severe, Canadian health managers are watching to see if American federal approval will be given to the Oregon Plan. That would set a precedent, not just as a possible plan of action, but as a process. One can anticipate that such a shift may follow in Canada.

How the Individual Might Pay for Services Beyond the Universal Medicare Package

There are a number of excellent and innovative ideas for how people might pay for the services not available within a basic medicare package. These include, among other things, a lottery system, a registered health-benefit savings plan and supplementary insurance.

The lottery for rare, expensive services for which demand exceeds supply,, might be similar to the current U.S. Immigration lottery. Applicants are selected randomly for immigration when the flow is too great. Such random selection (similar to a jury selection) would govern access for limited supply services such as esoteric transplants.

The registered health-benefit savings plan (RHBSP) for medical services anticipated at a future time would be similar to a retirement savings plan. If everyone is likely to want a particular health service at a certain time in the future (rather than it being a random event) then one must plan for it like a child's college education fund. You could save for your heart transplant in advance.

Way out speculation about some of these potentially desirable ficticious items can be found in the writings of William Gibson. His novel *Neuromancer* is a multiple-award winning book published in 1984 which was followed in 1986 by another novel, *Count Zero*. Gibson has become somewhat of a science-fiction, cyberpunk, cult in the world of artificial reality and virtual reality. Some of the leading graphics and other visualization software design gurus in North America utilize Gibson's ideas.

Neuromancer takes place in the near future where incredible medical advances have made possible all kinds of transplants, prosthetics (artificial devices such as robotic arms, etc.) and specifically a type of brain surgery which installs a socket into the skull and brain wired to your nervous system. This allows individuals to become instant experts – pilots, doctors, rocket scientists, cyberspace network users – by simply plugging a read-only-memory (ROM) chip into the socket behind the ear! The ROM chip has all the distilled expertise and wisdom of a particular specialist stored in its memory!

Because there are so many medical services in this fictional future, one has to have many levels of medical insurance coverage to get access to the huge variety of weird and wonderful things available. If one does not have such multi-layered coverage, there is also a huge black market in medical services. Most of these illicit biotech clinics are in the Far East. The point in all this is that so many things will be possible in ten to twenty years that we cannot currently conceive of them let alone plan to pay for them from a single restrictive health insurance plan. We need financial mechanisms similar to our retirement planning techniques.

Private insurance or publicly administered supplementary insurance as an add-on to provincial medicare could cover those services that have been removed from the government plan. People might be covered either by individual insurance policies (ie: Blue Cross Travel Insurance) or as part of employer-provided benefits packages.

Many critics make the point that optional multiple third party insurance packages, or other payment mechanisms that become part of the system, will add costs in the form of layers of overhead. According to some analysts, the U.S. could save $50-250 billion annually if such layers were removed. It really is not that simple. However, this unchecked multiplication of management cost is not inevitable in the Canadian system. Optional packages might be provided and billed largely by the provincial systems, avoiding the mistakes that have led to the American health services nightmare.

We must remember that we already have a multiple-layered system of care. Blue Cross and other "supplementary medical plans" pay for semi-private care in hospitals while drug and dental plans are common. But the costs of these plans, while rising, seem to be holding to reasonable levels. Some of these packages may be purchased by individual subscribers but most are available to those fortunate enough to be working for large companies or the government-funded sector. The plans are either part of their wage package or are provided on a partial funding basis as a tax benefit. The worrying aspect is that they are NOT generally available to the quickly growing numbers of people in the Burger King economy, the low-paying service related or part-time jobs, creating a very great inequity amongst Canadians even as governments in Canada boast of our "universal system".

Canada Needs a New Health System Vision: A Strategic Plan

To get to where we want to be with our reformed health system, in a realistic time frame, we must have a vision of something that is a genuine improvement over the excellent one we are losing. My vision of such a system is simple. The system must be more resilient in the face of inevitable cyclical economic fluctuations. It should be as lean and waste free as possible. This health system must be viewed as a vast and vital economic engine that can carry us into the far future. Ideally, it should be different from our current one, in that in addition to delivering good healthcare, it must also create and environment in which Innovation is King.

Healthcare innovators must be amply rewarded, whether their contributions are novel products or services that can be sold, or simply novel informational contributions to the health system. Only if this succeeds will the system contribute to more stability by the creation of spin-off economic opportunities for Canadians.

Our vision must include looking at every single aspect of healthcare as an opportunity to innovate to create new and better quality services and products that can be used at home and sold abroad. That is a tall order.

Japanese and German economic strategic planners adopt longer time frames than we do in North America, within which to design their long term goals. Matsushita (Panasonic) has plans for TWO HUNDRED YEARS from now. We must change. A single four or five year term of office for a government in Canada is not sufficient compared to the time that technical innovations take to diffuse into the marketplace. Typically, a pharmaceutical companies well understand, it may take ten years to bring a new drug to market. The biotechnology industry, which got its start in the early Eighties, is just now beginning to make money. Our economic institutions must somehow become the bridge which overcomes the gaps between the short economic and political cycles.

Similarly, advanced technology innovations in physics, chemistry, solid state electronics (microchips, etc.) take as long to become new consumer products. Laser physics brought us compact disc music players but they took more than a decade to take off. They have since become one of the most successful consumer electronics products in history. As well, the VCR took almost twenty years to develop from refrigerator-sized technology to the tiny camcorders and home VCRs of today. In every one of these success stories, there was risk, persistence, mistakes, and disappointment. There are no guarantees in building new enterprises in health or other market sectors.

Professor Jane Fulton of the University of Ottawa recently participated in an "electronic" town hall meeting hosted by Phil Donahue on U.S. television. She was the one Canadian representative amongst a panel of American health experts. What really irked me while watching and rewatching this program was Dr. Fulton's standing up and proclaiming that Canadians are content to be mediocre when it comes to healthcare. She does not speak for me or many others.

How are we going to compete with these countries if we continue our narrow-minded view of nation-building? Canada and Canadians had better start changing their attitudes to risk and long term planning or we are finished as a nation. Not only must our planning be very long range, but our national attitude to risk must be reinvented. Every good business planner and scientist knows that to get a successful product usually requires TEN, TWENTY, or more failures. You cannot design a successful product at one go in the market. All one can do is experiment over and over until success is achieved. Government must encourage an atmosphere that understands that most new innovational product attempts will fail! This requires risk capital. This requires tax benefits that are very appealing to risk capital. Without this attitude, we might as well forget any future dreams of a restructured Canadian economy let alone an even partly self-financing healthcare industry.

The Role of Government

Government needs to play a pivotal role in three specific areas as we build a future for our healthcare system. The first of these is standard setting; the second is quality assurance; and the third is an industrial strategy that recognizes the potential role of healthcare as a wealth generator.

Standards

With regard to standards, no Canadian looks with other than fear at the prospect of Canada further disintegrating into a federation of ten or twelve separate mini-states. The federal government should not abrogate all of its responsibilities in healthcare to ten or twenty very unequal provinces. It should be using national resources to take national initiatives to ensure that medical coverage is comparable, (and benefits are "portable" province to province). It should also be taking the lead in developing national standards of care and national health information systems as we discussed in Chapter 13.

Quality Assurance

The government's role in quality assurance is equally important. Medicare should ideally pay only for services which have been demonstrated scientifically to be efficacious or necessary. This should be the only criteria for consideration. As has been noted earlier in this book, probably less than 5% of all the things medicine currently does have been subjected to this kind of scrutiny. Not only physicians' services, but the services provided by every type of health professional, as well as non-medical alternatives, must be judged by the same rules. The result would be medical coverage that would be at least not ineffective or wasteful.

Industrial Strategy

The third major role for government is in the development of an industrial strategy. We have confronted a lot of jargon in this book such a effective, efficacious, constraint, reallocation, ration, manage and conserve. Most relate to the economic and operational problems of Medicare and other health systems. Most government solutions involve constraint, greater bureaucratic control, rationing, reducing, or shrinking services and finding ways to force or convince physicians to practice more cost effective medicine. Nowhere in any of the endless numbers of books and articles describing current problems has anyone recognized the fabulous opportunity this insatiable demand for health services offers to our economy.

Recently governments, both in Ontario and federally, have finally begun to at least sound like they understand what the country needs to reinvigorate its entrepreneurism. Ontario's new Industrial Policy, announced in July 1992, states that it "is about providing a framework that enables all segments of business, labour and government to work together as partners. It also is a way to ensure that government support for industrial development is strategic. It builds on the foundation of a market economy and on an appreciation of the important role that competition plays in innovation."

The new Ontario approach aims at working not with specific companies but with whole economic sectors to improve their competitiveness. If the government can be convinced that healthcare is a viable wealth producing sector, then some of the commitment to the policy and maybe some of the financial investment will be forthcoming. It is perhaps significant that among the specific accomplishments recognized in the policy publication at least two were healthcare related. One concerned the development by Toronto's Studio Innova of a CPR training manikin, the ACTRAR 911. The simple design of the manikin makes it 10 to 30 times less expensive than previous units. The second item mentioned was the establishment of the Toronto Biotechnical Initiative (TBI). This is a network of more than a hundred members of the Greater Toronto Area biotechnical community who have joined in an effort to increase the role of the area as a leading commercial and research centre for biotechnology.

A further encouraging message about healthcare emerges from the Ontario government's paper on its new industrial policy. It indicates that for the first time the Ministry of Health, not traditionally engaged in economic development efforts, would be included in sector strategies.

While the *Toronto Star* felt that the Ontario government was on the right track, it cautioned that to be effective, any provincial industrial strategy also depends on a strong federal role. So it is also encouraging that in the discussion paper issued by the Ottawa government concerning their proposed "Prosperity Initiative" that a number of important things have been recognized. The federal government admits that "investment in research and development (R & D) by Canadian private sector does not match investment by the private sector in other leading industrial nations." The federal discussion paper also says that it is important to use government investments in the most effective way and that "a domestic marketplace that encourages competition and innovation will promote long-term productivity and that means a better chance to compete globally."[1]

Since an enormous portion of both federal and provincial funds are invested in medicare, it would seem logical to make the most of that investment. And since the domestic market for health services is large and secure, what better place to encourage the competition and innovation that will help us compete internationally? It is likely that when the final federal report on "Prosperity Initiatives" is presented, it will include a competitiveness council that may further recognize the potential of healthcare as a growth industry.

Ways Governments Can Assist Canadian Healthcare Innovators

The past decade has seen a reaction against government involvement in encouraging and financing private business. The troubles of Novatel and the Alberta Heritage Fund stand as a warning, as if one was needed. And yet, there is no way, given our geography, population, and past history, that Canadian industry can compete globally without some very well thought out governmental assistance. It worked for the Japanese and surely we have learned enough (through hard experience) that we can make it work for us.

Hopefully, a healthy portion of the three year, $150 million Sector Partnership Fund will be allocated to developing the business potential of the healthcare sector. While the intent of the Ontario government seems admirable, they must realize that just "clearing the path for business success" isn't enough. Aspiring and innovative new companies need start-up capital and operating credit to bridge them over their R&D phase. Whether we like it or not, governments in Canada have long played a role in providing or encouraging the provision of this kind of capital. It is one thing to put $930 million into a job creation fund and $1.1 billion into another training program, as Ontario is doing, but we must consider *what* jobs we are training people for. Government funds must be allocated towards the fostering of the innovation that will allow the creation of new marketable products and services. Experience has shown that it is successful small to medium sized companies who develop new business that are the greatest creators of new jobs.

It may seem that I'm arguing that governments back off from healthcare, on the one hand, and then arguing that they jump back in, on the other. In fact, that is exactly what I am suggesting. The best role for government is not in monopolizing healthcare delivery, but encouraging innovation and entrepreneurism. As Ontario's Industrial Policy states itself, "no government can create wealth or increase value added on its own."

There are a number of specific ways that healthcare could benefit from strategic government encouragement. One of these is in the medical application of computer software. Canada could excel here. As I pointed out in Chapter 13, medical records and case management; a national health information utility network; and a drug therapy database, are just some of the applications which Canadians could develop. We have the computer programming expertise and we have a healthcare system in place that is of a small enough size and has a degree of sophistication that would make computerization manageable. A Canadian software expert committee would ascertain in the short-term which kinds of applications will advance the science of medical computing, and fund the most promising ideas with incentives for software developers.

Such a proposed committee could involve representatives from the Medical Research Council of Canada (MRC) and perhaps the Canadian Institute for Advanced Research. Over the years, the MRC role has been primarily as a funding body for biomedical research in Canada. The role has been largely reactive, relying on Canada's scientists to submit projects. The MRC has never undertaken research, unlike the U.S. National Institutes of Health in Bethseda, Maryland, where there is a large NIH research community. Currently, the MRC, under its new president, Dr. Henry Friesen, believes the MRC should play a leadership role and wants the council to develop a strategic, long-term plan of action. I believe this new perspective is complimentary to an involvement both in basic medical science, as well as in the software engineering, which will be crucial to future advances in both clinical and medical research.

As well, we must involve more pragmatic computer experts from the private sector: The voice of the marketplace must draw closer to the academic medical community just as it is doing in the educational sector.

The Scientific Research Tax Credit system was abolished by the federal government a few years ago as a result of abuses. It has been replaced by the Scientific Research and Experimental Development Tax Credit (SR&ED) which is much more effective and user friendly. The new program allows a company to receive tax credits, or tax refunds, if their profits are not high, for up to 35% of what they invest in bonafide research. The plan is administered by Revenue Canada, and while the accounting for the tax credit is suitably scrutinized, there is no requirement to have projects reviewed by outside panels or bureaucrats. If a company is spending its own money on R&D and can account for it, that is good enough for the tax man. Along with Ontario's Medical Innovation Fund and such programs as Small Business Development Corporations Loans, it is possible for an entrepreneur to cobble together a support package to allow the development of new ideas. But a tremendous amount of energy is diverted from research by this requirement to chase funding. The Ontario government's efforts to consolidate the offices that administer various programs is therefore a welcome announcement. The question remains as to whether enough is being done to stimulate innovation.

What Have We Learned From the Old System

The fading old paradigm of Medicare has many parallels in the moral of the best-selling book *The Bonfire of the Vanities*, a tale of greed and pride consuming and then transforming the lives of a number of upscale New Yorkers. In the old undimensional Canadian health system, everyone has had everything they wanted, on demand, and from a single source. It is turning out that this approach is neither practical, equitable, nor affordable.

Government must get out of the business of limiting and controlling in its dealings with healthcare, and into the business of inspiring the participants and stakeholders. We are all on the same side. In summary, what we need is:

- **A Basic Package of Essential and Effective Services:** much leaner and meaner, learning from the excesses and wasteful experiences of the past. Equity means fair, not identical. It is not equitable to provide the same thing to everyone; there must be Choice. The package must be comprehensive, but within society's ability to pay. It must be accessible to all, portable, no matter where you live in Canada. The principles of non-profit public administration of Medicare must be preserved.

- **Democratic Process:** We cannot restructure and rebuild our healthcare system without consultation and open and wide-ranging public debate. There are three "players": The payers (governments, representing us all as taxpayers); the public (including advocacy groups): and healthcare providers. (No one said it would be easy!)

- **Choice:** Technology is creating and will increasingly create new opportunities to deliver more and better health products and services to consumers. The future of healthcare must be based on choice. All kinds of layers or enhancements beyond the basic health benefits package must be available as options, with a mix of public and private, profit and non-profit providers, expanding on the current system.

- **Healthcare that is perceived as an integral part of a Canadian Industrial and Economic Long Range Strategy:** It is an essential part of the economic engine of present and future economies.

- **A Canadian National Health Information Utility:** This must become an immediate priority. Funding must be allocated nationally. The system must be viewed in all its aspects as a potentially saleable and exportable product. Every doctor's office, clinic, community health facility, hospital, nursing home, and alternative care facility must use it; every place people receive care must have a computer that people can utilize to access the system. Public access must be assured. This system will empower ALL users, consumers and providers.

- **Research and Development:** In basic health sciences, health service delivery, operational methods, and medical application, software must be supported far beyond current levels. Every aspect of healthcare must be perceived as an opportunity to innovate and create marketable products and services for Canadian and other markets. The diffusion of new technologies from such activities must flow as rapidly as possible to Canadian entrepreneurs.

- **To address morale problems in the health provider system:** Better health provider's job security and compensation. Whether alternative payment methods (salary) evolve or not, there must be many more paid opportunities for fellowships, continued education, sabbaticals, and learning experiences for people at all levels in the profession. There must be more rotations, mobility, and flexibility in medical experiences. Innovation must be stimulated, expected, and rewarded at every level.

I believe these principles can enrich and inspire all participants to create a different, more responsive, and better system. It will remain for those people we elect and those we pay to come up with the detailed blueprints for action and to implement the changes agreed to.

Conclusion

This book was motivated by the belief that modern medical science, with all its past and present triumphs, is just beginning to discover itself. The book of current medical practice is daily rewritten. Every day, physicians face patients with an unbelievable lack of awareness of the critical information published, information they have not yet heard about that might positively affect the outcome of their particular problems. They do this unknowingly, and because of the impossibility for any human to be aware of, let alone absorb, all of the information that is so rapidly uncovered in this Fourth Wave.

The single most important event in all of earth's 4 billion years of biological evolution is now unfolding. The unlocking of the genetic code or script. It may take ten years, or fifty. We are about to become the children of the book of life, and as we learn to read it, we will eventually tamper with it and ultimately rewrite it.

Faced with the full implications of this event, only one inescapable conclusion exists about the future of human health, and health systems. It is intertwined with information. Healthcare futures, and health futures, are also an information future. Only one single best way exists to provide the public with effective and affordable healthcare. It is to build a system around the flow of information. Information that empowers both caregivers and care receivers.

The paradigm for the health system in the immediate term, as well as the more distant future, must include powerful information systems at the centre and at the most remote user level. We must provide both patients and their healthcare professionals with the information about what is possible and what is effective at any particular moment. This will enable the providers to do their best at any given intervention. It will also help to relieve and inform anxious patients about the best treatment they can expect at any given moment, rather than chase after fraudulent and elusive remedies.

There is much opportunity here. We had better get on with building such a system as soon as possible.

APPENDIX A

A Better Way to Gauge Fees is to Base Them on Experience

Reprinted with permission of the editor, from *The Medical Post*, November 12, 1991.

Of all the many failings of the present restrictive situation prevalent in Canada regarding compensation for doctors in private practice, to me the most frustrating is the lack of any room for rewarding the expertise and experience of the practitioner.

The practitioner who has grown and matured in knowledge and clinical experience after a number of years is restricted – by law – to charging exactly the same per procedure as the person who just graduated and started practice today.

That runs counter to common sense. It is an abomination. It doesn't apply anywhere else in normal business and economic life, and interestingly enough the very governments that have proposed and enacted such nonsense are themselves very much tied into all sorts of progressive compensatory scales.

The absence of any reward for experience and excellence acts as a profound disincentive that eventually corrodes away any interest on the part of individuals to keep current with their knowledge base, with new advances, and with the upkeep of their own offices and equipment. If you get exactly the same for doing the "minimum" as for doing better, then why bother to do better?

All the evidence, and it is enormous, suggests that in the absence of incentives, people eventually just do not bother. "Self-respect" may keep some people going for a while – and this is what is happening here in Canada – but eventually all but a very small minority let their standards drop.

The inevitability of that outcome appears to be a psychological truism of human nature, and I am aware of absolutely no evidence that would suggest the NDP or any other group has the slightest prospect of changing human nature. One of Dr. Martin Barkin's greatest deficiencies as deputy minister of health in Ontario was his inability to appreciate this. The blatant decline in quality of service, which is being widely commented on, is one of the most damning features of his legacy.

Britain has tried a system of "merit" awards and when the Liberal-NDP coalition a few years ago restricted the rights of doctors to bill patients appropriately, it was widely quoted that then Ontario premier David Peterson had expressed some interest in this approach. My understanding, though, of the British experience is that it didn't work well, that it aroused enormous hostilities and resentments between those who were acknowledged and those who were not, and that the process was too secretive and appeared to be highly arbitrary.

It would be very difficult, especially with a smaller population of physicians, to make anonymous evaluations and decide who is deserving. It would be very difficult to decide who would do the selection. Would it be someone from the bureaucracy? If so, how are they – nonmedical people – going to judge? Would it be medical personnel? But then who? Would those in private practice feel comfortable with senior academics doing the choosing? I wouldn't. The understanding that senior academics have of the finer points of private practice, and of the priorities and approaches of practice, is often limited. How were they going to judge? What would be their criteria? Who would make clinical judgements, or would we have academic criteria deciding clinical excellence?

But equally fraught with complications would be leaving such decisions in the hands of those from your local medical society or regulatory college. Again, what criteria are they going to use? The possibilities of personal favoritism, of extraclinical factors in terms of personal acquaintance, work on committees, referrals, even reports from patients or paramedical staff that may be based on questionable criteria would all have too many subjective factors and be too open to bias to be effective.

I have come to the conclusion that rewarding excellence is too difficult, and poses too many potential problems and inequities. I am therefore going to make the simpler suggestion that we reward experience instead.

I am proposing that for each five-year period from the time the physician started practice there be a 7% increment in their fee per procedure. I suggest this 7% increase above the baseline fee (the OHIP or other provisional rates "negotiated" each year between government and those who are supposed to act on behalf of doctors) continue for each five-year period until the physician reaches the age of 60 when it stops.

On that basis – assuming a minimum age of starting college at 18, medical school at 20, graduating at 24, and completing either a family practice residency at 27 or a specialty residency at 29 – there would be a maximum of six increments. The final level the senior physician would end up with would be a fee that is 42% higher per procedure than the fee the beginner receives, at the base level, a difference that I do not think is out of line with comparable differences in government, business or other economic areas.

The main objection to this is that some people do not progress over the years, and that such a scheme might allow some doctors to do nothing other than just fill out the time, knowing they will get their increase with age.

To counteract this, I would suggest that certain criteria be fulfilled to receive this increment. Such criteria might include annual certified attendance and participation at recognized and appropriate courses, a certain amount of teaching, similar academic work demonstrating continuing progress, or the publication of contributions to the literature.

With the addition of such criteria, there would be far fewer people who would "slip through the cracks." What little is lost by a small number receiving the increment without really deserving it is more than compensated for by the fact that with such an incentive most doctors, as they mature, would feel they were being compensated for their increased understanding and experience in at least some minimal way.

No one questions the brightness and enthusiasm of youth, and that new graduates are often in closer touch with new techniques and technologies, and newer diagnostic approaches. But so often the best clinical decision still requires the maturity and experience that only comes with time.

I don't expect these proposals to be adopted by those who "officially" negotiate fees on behalf of doctors. I do not believe they have the intention, the insight, the foresight, or the capability of thinking in these terms. I have absolutely zero confidence in such a negotiating team as the one that left Ontario physicians with such a disastrous recent agreement. I don't know the situation well enough regarding negotiations in the other provinces.

I think a more productive approach for those who think these proposals have merit is to campaign through your parliamentary representatives, to persuade the government that such a system would be in the best interests of the public in providing an incentive system that will enable doctors to maintain some enthusiasm in the present restrictive system.

– *Dr. Joseph Berger, Toronto, Toronto, Ont.*

Are We being Asked to Practise Ideology Instead of Medicine?

Reprinted with permission of the editor, from *The Medical Post*, November 19, 1991.

Once in a while, for my sins, I still must read government reports, and once in a while sifting through the dross still yields nuggets of information. The latest tome to thump on my desk is the report to the deputy ministers of health, our real bosses, "Toward Integrated Medical Resource Policies in Canada."

It is about us doctors; how we should be trained, how many of us there should be, where we should practice, how many of us should be specialists. There is not much bread in it, and little that is new, but one clause did leap at me from the page. Despite its length, it deserves quoting in full, and discusssing in depth.

#10, p. 3-3. There is a continuing evolution from the view of physicians as the private agents for their patients and their own interests, to the view of physicians as clinically skilled agents serving the collective goals of a publicly funded healthcare system. Physicians, more than any other group in Canadian society, have rights and privileges that allow them to satisfy professional interests within a publicly funded enterprise.

This system of "private participants in a public enterprise" requires the reconciliation of "professional" and "political" ideologies concerning both the content and context of medicine. Progress in this direction, which has been slowly evolving since the inception of "Medicare" may be aided by means of additional incentives that make the accountability of physicians to collective public objectives more explicit.

The more often and more closely I read it, the worse it sounds. The CMA has a Code of Ethics which starts off quite simply, "Consider first the well-being of the patient." Most of us still subscribe to this; that when the chips are down, what matters is the physician's responsibility to the single individual in his/her care.

Most of the old simplicities are long gone – we are all members of health-care teams, and patients do not pay us directly for their own care. What care we can offer them is very often determined by others. But the buck does stop here, in the ultimate, one-on-one, relationship and responsibility.

This is a very long way from the physician as "an agent serving the goals of a publicly funded healthcare system." Canadians have decided on such a system; they have not totally subordinated the individual to it, nor have they required that the physician consider first the system rather than the patient.

The relationship between the individual and the system is being worked out, slowly and painfully, as it has been borne in upon us that fair promises, "All we want to do is pay the doctors," are glib falsehoods and pots of fairy gold at the end of Rainbow Reports. The moral physician considers the system within which we work and its resources, as finite, to be used rationally and carefully.

But the individual doctor cannot be the gatekeeper for the individual patient, rationing care by considering the system first and the individual thereafter. Putting the physician in such a moral dilemma can have varied results, none of them good.

One is the purely utilitarian evaluation of the patient as the servant of the state, the bee in the hive; is he, in that context, "worth" saving? An alternative is to erect a structure of false values, pretending that the doctor's personal estimates of a patient's worth to society are in fact made on objective, medical criteria, as British physicians are said to have done, when choosing who would receive treatment for end stage renal failure.

Predictably, the poor, the brown, the ill-educated and the inarticulate fared worse than the rich, the white, the learned and the domineering.

"Reconciliation of professional and political ideologies" sounds a difficult balancing act, taking into account the very recent political upheavals in some provinces. The political ideology changed radically in my own Saskatchewan in October 21 with the provincial election.

Should my medical practice swing like a weathervane into the wind of conformity?

Is my ability as a doctor to be valued by how well and how quickly I can make that change, like the doubleplusgood duckspeaker in *1984* whose erstwhile enemies became in a moment allies, and vice-versa? There are some things I cannot in conscience reconcile myself with, and quite a few of them are political.

The authors of the report believe we are slowly evolving in this direction, and we can explain this on either Lamarckian or Darwinian theories. They would like it to be quicker; it may be "aided by incentives that make the accountability of physicians to public objectives more explicit."

This sounds very much like, "We have ways of making you conform," spoken in a strong guttural. So-called public objectives are most often the ideas of politicians, given shape and substance by civil servants. On the rare occasions on which the Canadian public are invited to comment upon them, they seem oddly unappreciative, "Take the politics out of Medicare" is a recurrent theme.

When the citizens of Oregon were asked to rank their healthcare objectives explicitly in order, those upon which they put the highest priority were quite different from those, so far as we can perceive them because they are mostly unstated, of Canadian Medicare. The Canadian public are not Oregonians, and might have a different order of rank values, but they have not been asked to state them.

The whole clause smells very bad indeed. We are way beyond looking for communists under the bed, or Nazis in the closet, but it has a nasty feel of the 1930s. The overwhelming problem of Medicare is healthcare rationing – if the pie is too small for all the demands for slices to be met, how do we decide who gets what – who decides, on what moral grounds of value, and on what authority?

This has to be done somewhere, somehow, by someone, but the person and the place and the time are not the individual doctor and patient in their unique relationship. Practising with a true regard for limited public resources is one thing; making individual judgments of value on patients is quite another, and this inescapably seems to be what this clause suggests. I hope that few of us would practise in accord with someone else's "political ideologies." This is not what Medicare was meant to be about.

– *Dr. Harry Emson, Saskatoon, Saskatchewan*

ENDNOTES

Introduction

1. "Laughren says Ontario to limit medical services," "The Ontario government is planning limits on some medical services to slow the growth of the health-care budget," *The Globe and Mail*, December 20, 1991.
2. "Porter's study takes a chilling look at our competitive failings," *Financial Times of Canada*, October 28, 1991.

Chapter 1

1. "Biotech: America's Dream Machine. Will it become the dominant growth industry of the 1990's?" "By the year 2000 according to several forecasts, $50 billion worth of biotech products should be on sale around the globe." *BusinessWeek*, March 2, 1992.
2. Davies, *The Matter Myth*.

Chapter 2

1. "Silver threads threaten to strangle the system," *The Globe and Mail*, May 1, 1992.

Chapter 3

1. Oregon Health Services Commission, *Prioritization of Health Services*.
2. I've based this chapter on articles by Dr. A. McPherson and Dr. Harry E. Emson, in the *Canadian Medical Association Journal* 1991; 145 (11), and reproduce some of their thoughts without particular attribution, with permission. "Down the Oregon Trail: The Way for Canada?" Harry E. Emson, MD, FRCP, and "The Oregon Plan: Rationing in a Rational Society," A. McPherson, MD, PhD.

Chapter 4

1. Kanouse, *Changing Medical Practice Through Technology Assessment*.

Chapter 5

1. Professor Jane Fulton, Health Policy, University of Ottawa. *Morningside* discussion, CBC, September 1991.

Chapter 6

1. "Don't make MD's 'cost-containment' agents," Robert Veatch, *Family Practice*, December 7, 1991.
2. "A Different View of Queues in Ontario," Dr. David Naylor, *Health Affairs*, Fall, 1991.
3. "Smartcard Software Glitch Delays Pilot Project." *The Financial Post*, November 27, 1991.
4. Kanouse, *Changing Medical Practice Through Technology Assessment*.
5. Israelson, "Not so pretty in pink."
6. Editorial, "Suntan lotion and the cost of Medicare."
7. Editorial, "How many doctors is too many?"
8. Masayuki Ikuma Suzuki, *The Globe and Mail, Report on Business*, March, 1992.

Chapter 7

1. Reuters, "French health care workers denounce national system," *The Globe and Mail*, November 18, 1991.
2. Jocelyne Zablit, "France's festering health-care wound," *The Globe and Mail*, November 18, 1991.
3. "Removal of Electrolysis from OHIP Fee Schedule," *The Globe and Mail*, October 3, 1991. (In effect, November 15, 1991.)

Chapter 8

1. McNinch, "Hospital crisis, low FP input may be linked."
2. "Capitation: more costly than fee-for-service?" Review of an article in *BMJ* which suggests HOMOx are more expensive than fee-for-service. *Family Practice*, August 4, 1990.
3. "Joint Management Committee Update," *Ontario Medical Review*, November, 1991.
4. "B.C. Report advises beds, fees be limited," *The Medical Post*, November 26, 1991.
5. Barer, *Toward Integrated Medical Resource Policies for Canada*.
6. Lowry, Fran, *Many Quebec MDs search for greener pastures as morale of province's doctors nosedives*, Special Report, *Canadian Medical Association Journal*, 1991; 145(4), 329-332.
7. "Shortage Looms," *The Medical Post*, January 21, 1992.
8. Canadian Press, "Quebec tackles health costs," *The Globe and Mail*, December 18, 1991. Contenta, Sandro, "Quebec health fee plan is panned," *The Toronto Star*, December 22, 1991.
9. "One way to cut health costs," *The Financial Post*, November 7, 1991.

Chapter 10

1. Comments by Dr. Richard Goldbloom, Chairman of the Canadian Taskforce on the Periodic Health Exam, and Professor of Pediatrics, Dalhousie University:

    "Ever since the Lalonde report on the future of health care, we've all had this idea that by spending more money on prevention, we'll save money on treatment – unfortunately, there's just no evidence to support that idea."

    "It's a misrepresentation for government or the medical establishment to tell the public that preventive care saves money... It will probably cost more money."

    "Most preventive interventions after childhood cost more money than they save, with a few exceptions, such as smoking cessation."

2. Frame, P.S., "A critical review of adult health maintenance." *Journal of Family Practice*, 1986; 22(6): 511-520.
3. Satenstein, "Prevention in Family Practice..."

Chapter 11

1. "Government hiding health care spending cuts: Conference." *Family Practice*, November 16, 1991.

Chapter 13

1. "PORT confirms one clinical impression and offers some surprises about relative outcomes." *Ophthalmology*, June, 1991, 895-902.

Chapter 14

1. Toffler, *The Third Wave*, p. 131.
2. "Needless Needles," *Time*, July 6, 1992. Sandia National Labs is developing a similar product.
3. "3-D Human Anatomical Database," *Computer Graphics World*, December 1991.
4. Barbour et. al., "Imaging of Subsurface Regions of Random Media by Remote Sensing," *SPIE*, Vol. 1431, 1991.

Chapter 15

1. *Prosperity Through Competetiveness,* Prosperity Secretariat, Government of Canada, 1991.

BIBLIOGRAPHY

Books

Barsky, Arthur. *Worried Sick: Our Troubled Quest for Wellness*, Little, Brown and Co., 1988.

Begin, Monique. *Medicare: Canada's Right to Health*, Optimum Publishing International, Montreal, 1988.

Bishop, J. E., and M. Waldholz. *Genome: The story of the most astonishing scientific adventure of our time – the attempt to map all the genes in the human body*, Simon & Schuster, New York, 1990.

Burke, T., and G. Dolf, et al., eds. *DNA Fingerprinting: Approaches and Applications*, Springer Verlag, Boston, Berlin, 1991.

Crommelin, P. J., and M. Schellekens, eds. *From Clone to Clinic*, Kluwer Academic Publishers, 1990.

Cumper, George E. *The Evaluation of National Health Systems*, Oxford University Press, London, 1991.

Davies, Paul and John Gribbin. *The Matter Myth*, Simon & Schuster, New York, 1992.

Drexler, Eric, Peterson, Chris, and Gayle Pergamit. *Unbounding the Future: The Nanotechnology Revolution*, Morrow, New York, 1991.

Federoff, Sergey, et al, ed. *Atherosclerosis: Cellular and Molecular Interactions in the Artery Wall*, Plenum Press, New York, 1991.

Fettner, Ann Giudici. *Viruses: Agents of Change*, McGraw-Hill, New York, 1990.

Gilder, George. *Microcosim, The Quantum Revolution in Economics and Technology*, Simon & Schuster, New York, 1989.

Hall, Mark and John Barry. *Sunburst: The Ascent of Sun Microsystems*, Contemporary Books, 1990.

Hausser, K.H., and H. R. Kalbitzer. *NMR in Medicine & Biology: Structure Determination in Tomography, In-vivo Spectroscopy*, Springer-Verlag, New York, Berlin, 1991.

Ilich, Ivan. *Limits to Medicine: Medical Nemesis: The Expropriation of Health*, McClelland and Stewart, Toronto, 1976.

Kanouse, David E., et al. *Changing Medical Practice Through Technology Assessment, An Evaluation of the NIH Consensus Development Program*, The Rand Corporation, Health Administration Press, 1989.

Maxmem, Jerrold S. MD. *The Post-Physician Era: Medicine in the Twenty-First Century*, Wiley, New York, 1976.

Ornish, Dean, MD. *Dr. Dean Ornish's Program for Reversing Heart Disease Without Surgery*, Random House, New York, 1990.

Pastorino, Ugo, and K.H. Waun, eds. *Chemoimmuno Prevention of Cancer*, Thieme Medical Publishers, Inc., New York, 1991.

Rachlis M. and C. Kushner. *Second Opinion: What's Wrong with Canada's Health Care System and How to Fix It*, Toronto, 1988.

Sagan, Leonard A. *The Health of Nations: True Causes of Sickness and Well-being*, Basic Books, New York, 1987.

Shapiro, Robert, MD. *The Human Blueprint: The Race to Unlock the Secrets of Our Genetic Script*, St. Martin's Press, New York, 1991.

Spilker, R. and M. Friedman, ed. *1991 Biomechanics Symposium*, The American Society of Mechanical Engineers, AMD-Vol. 120, New York, 1991.

Spurgeon, Peter, ed. *The Changing Face of the National Health Service in the 1990's*, Longman, London, 1990.

Toffler, Alvin. *The Third Wave*, Bantam Books, New York, 1980.
Verna, Roberto, et al, ed. *Bioengineered Molecules: Basic and Clinical Aspects*, Raven Press, New York, 1989.
Wehrli, Felix W. *Fast-Scan Magnetic Resonance: Principles and Applications*, Raven Press, New York, 1990.
Wilcox, Lewis DeWitt, M.D. *Where Is My Doctor?* Fitzhenry & Whiteside, Toronto, 1977.

Articles

"Biotech: America's Dream Machine. Will it become the dominant growth industry of the 1990's?" *BusinessWeek*, March 2, 1992.
Burstyn, Varda, "Making Perfect Babies," *The Canadian Forum*, April 1992.
Corcoran, Terence, "Medicare's incurable illness: it can't work," *The Globe and Mail*, November 23, 1991.
– "Why are our doctors leaving?" *The Globe and Mail*, ROB, April 3, 1992.
Dunlop, Marilyn, "Prescription for Ontario's ailing hospitals, Attention to quality can cut costs former health ministry official says," *The Toronto Star*, December 11, 1991.
Faltermayer, Edmund, "Let's *Really* Cure the Health System," *Fortune Magazine*, March 23, 1992.
"The Gene Doctors Roll Up Their Sleeves," *BusinessWeek*, March 30, 1992.
Gibbon, Anne, "Quadra comes of age: B.C. firm's drug battles cancer," *The Globe and Mail*, April 20, 1992.
Heginbotham, Chris, "Rationing," *BMJ*, 1992; 301:496-9.
Hudson, Kellie, "Emerging case load a crap shoot," *The Toronto Star*, August 17, 1991.
Linton, Adam L., "Will healthcare need to be rationed?" *Ontario Medical Review*, January, 1992.
Mackie, Richard, "Ontario poised to cut some services," *The Globe and Mail*, December 5, 1991.
Matas, Robert, "Three NDP governments to unite against user fees," *The Globe and Mail*, February 15, 1992.
Mickleburgh, Rod, "CAC urges health care sacrifices: Consumer group says public must become cost-conscious in doctor's office," *The Globe and Mail*, January 24, 1992.
– "Silver threads threaten to strangle the system," *The Globe and Mail*, May 1, 1992.
"Removal of Electrolysis from OHIP Fee Schedule," *The Globe and Mail*, October 3, 1991.
Roberts, David, "Health care sales proposal attacked: Leaked Manitoba memo identifies possible services for sick Americans," *The Globe and Mail*, November 16, 1991.
Satenstein, G., MD, and J. Lemelin, MD et al., "Prevention in Family Practice, Consensus Statement from the Front Line," *Canadian Family Physician*, October, 1991.
Saunders, John, "Bush plan for health care aims to keep system private: Canadian model dismissed as cure worse than disease," *The Globe and Mail*, February 7, 1992.
Seidon, Howard, MD, "Executive medical checks overrated and unnecessary," *The Toronto Star*, October 3, 1991.
"Surgery Needed: A Survey of Health Care," *The Economist*, July 6, 1991.
Sweet, Lois, "The Hospital Squeeze," *The Toronto Star*, November 16, 1991.
Taylor, David, "Prescribing in Europe – forces for change," *BMJ*, 1992; 304:239-42.
Taylor, Paul, "Friendly video gives power to the patient," *The Globe and Mail*, April 30, 1992.
"The Tiniest Transplants," *The Economist*, April 25, 1992.
Walker, Michael, "Canadian Health Care is a Model for Disaster," *The Wall Street Journal*, October 18, 1991.

Weinkauf, Darrel J., and Gerald C. Rowland MD, "Patient Conditions at the Primary-Care Level: A Commentary on Resource Allocation," *Ontario Medical Review*, January, 1992.

Welch, H. Gilbert, "Should the Health Care Forest be Selectively Thinned by Physicians or Clear Cut by Payers?" *Annals of Internal Medicine*, Vol. 115, No. 3, August 1991, pp. 223-6.

Electronic Media

"Between the Lines," TVO Program. Guests: Ontario Health Minister, Francis Larkin; Dr. William Goodman, OMA Chairman; Dr. Tom Dickson, University of Saskatchewan; Professor Glen Beck, University of Saskatchewan.

"Condition Critical: American Healthcare Forum," Hosted by Phil Donahue, WGBH Boston Production, April 8, 1992.

"MacNeil Lehrer Report," Debate between Bob Rae, Premier of Ontario and Gail Wilensky, Deputy Assistant to George Bush for policy development, April 21, 1992.

"Morningside," CBC Radio – Medicare. Guests: Monique Begin, Former Minister of Health; Martin Barkin; Jane Fulton, Health Policy, University of Ottawa, September, 1991.

Government Publications

Barer, Morris L. and Greg L. Stodart, *Toward Integrated Medical Resource Policies for Canada*, Directorate, Health Services Branch, Health and Welfare Canada, 1991.

Barrows, D. *Ontario's International Competitiveness*, Ontario Centre For International Business, September, 1991.

British Columbia. *Ministry of Health, 1989/1990 Annual Report*, 1991.

Canada. *Medication and Health Policy: A Research Agenda*, Science Council of Canada, October 1991, Catalogue No. SS31-21/1991.

Canada. *Genetics in Canadian Health Care*, Science Council of Canada, 1991, Catalogue No. SS22-1991/42E.

Ontario Ministry of Health. *Information and Technology Strategic Plan*, April 1989.

Ontario Ministry of Health. *Deciding the Future of Our Health Care – An Overview For Public Discussion*, April 1989.

Ontario Ministry of Industry, Trade and Technology. *An Industrial Framework for Ontario*, July 1992.

Ontario Premier's Council On Health Strategy. *From Vision To Action*, Health Care System Committee, 1989.

Ontario. "Managing Health Care Resources: Meeting Ontario's Priorities," Supplementary Paper 1992 Ontario Budget, May 1992.

Ontario. *1992 Ontario Budget*, 1992.

Ontario. *Toward a Shared Direction For Health in Ontario*, Report of the Ontario Health Review Panel (Evans Committee), June, 1987.

Oregon Health Services Commission. *Prioritization of Health Services: A Report to the Governor and Legislature*, Office of Salem, Oregon, 1991.

Royal Commission on Health Care and Costs. *Closer to Home*, Justice Peter Seaton,

United States of America. *U.S. Departments of Health and Human Services Health Technology Assessment and Research Reports 1986-1991*, Agency for Health Care Policy and Research (AHCPR), 1991.

INDEX

abuse, 19, 95, 116, 122, 181
access, 162, 194
accountability, 150
Agency for Health Care Policy and Research (AHCPR), 166
AIDS, 33, 84, 115, 118, 170, 171
Alberta,
allergies, 142, 144
allergists, 144
alternative healers, 72, 116, 123, 128
Alzheimer's disease, 32, 145
American, 14, 15, 92, 98, 103, 125, 127, 129, 130, 144, 161, 169,
American, 175, 188
aneurysm, 132
antibodies, 172
antisense moloecules, 171
arresting CAD, 128
arthritis, 25, 142, 144
arthroscopic, 47, 166
assistive devices, 165
atherosclerosis, 25, 129, 130, 137
Barer-Stoddart Report, 77, 106, 107, 108
bed closures, 16
benefits packages, 186
biosensors, 178, 179
biotechnology, 27, 169, 170, 186, 188, 190
blame, 14, 16, 35, 30, 66, 134
blood pressure, 26, 34, 142, 144, 152, 179
breast cancer, 69, 115, 131, 177
breast biopsy, 19, 177
Britain, 25, 29, 44, 65, 74, 90, 98
British Columbia, 37, 83, 105, 117, 134, 135, 146, 161
Bulletin Board, 35, 161
bypass surgery, 91, 92, 128, 137
Canada, 11, 13, 15, 18, 21, 29, 32, 37, 40, 47, 50, 54, 62, 66, 70, 81, 90, 115, 133, 169, 175, 181, 184, 187, 192, 193
cancer, 24, 25, 26, 118, 122, 125, 131, 142, 144, 145, 158, 170, 173
cap, 14, 38, 51, 104, 106, 118
capitalism, 181
capitation, 98, 99
cardiovascular, 142, 144, 168
caring, 23, 24, 116, 117, 170

cataract, 164
catastrophic illness, 25, 48, 184
cell signalling, 171
change, 14, 184, 188
chip, 139, 140, 188
choice, 145, 184, 194
cholesterol, 26, 128, 135, 136, 137, 138, 143, 146, 174, 179
cholesterol-lowering agents, 128, 136
clawback, 104
clinical trials, 53, 179
commodity, 28
community health centre, 76, 78, 79, 94, 97, 99, 101, 124, 139, 145
compact disk (CD-ROM), 140, 167
competitive, 17, 155, 184, 190
computer, 11, 30, 155, 182
computer software, 57, 192
consensus, 67
consumerism, 26
coronary artery disease (CAD), 128, 168
cosmetic surgery, 57, 70, 91, 105, 185
cost saving, 141
cost-containment, 11, 154
cost-effective, 66, 67, 101, 103, 105, 159, 160, 164
cottage industry, 155
database, 35, 155, 161, 163, 164, 165, 167, 192
deficits, 94
deinsure, 39, 146, 149
delays, 69, 127
delisting, 142, 143, 154, 185
demand, 46, 133, 152, 190
deprenyl, 32
dermatologists, 45, 144, 150
despair, 24
diabetes, 26, 125, 131, 143, 144, 173
diagnostic, 148, 152
double-doctoring, 163
drug benefit, 37, 38, 137
drugs, 24
economy, 22
effectiveness, 41, 52, 57, 150, 166, 189, 194, 195, 196
electrolysis, 88, 144
emergency, 16, 95, 96, 102, 127, 139
enabling technologies, 174, 175

encounter, 15, 126, 138, 140, 141, 144, 154, 168
entitlement, 36, 50, 52
entrepreneurial, 11, 17, 86, 90, 93, 119, 183, 190, 192, 194
environmental, 36, 183
erythropoietin, 33, 171, 182
essential, 40, 41, 43, 47, 49, 164, 185, 194
European, 14, 169, 175
exercise, 165

family doctor, 96, 113, 144
fatigue, 123
fear, 153, 154, 189
fee-for-service, 22, 97, 101, 106, 145
fiscal responsibility, 29, 75, 152, 154, 181
Fourth Wave, 180, 195
Framingham Study, 125, 129
French, 84
gatekeeper, 51, 66, 75
genetic, 26, 58, 125, 129, 170, 172
genetic code, 27, 183, 195
genetic defects, 60, 131
German, 188
growth factors, 34, 182
growth hormone, 31, 32
guideline gap, 130, 166
guidelines, 53, 54, 127, 130, 147, 166

HDL-cholesterol, 136
HEAL, 50
healing, 24, 123
health policy shifts, 121
Health Insurance Number (HIN), 86, 118, 138
healthcare, 30, 58, 181, 183, 187, 189, 190, 193
heart attack, 20, 129, 130, 136, 137
heart disease, 25, 118, 131
high technology, 26, 147, 152, 169
home care, 64, 94, 158
hospital, 16, 28, 61
housecall, 86, 88

iatrogenic, 28, 30
imaging, 59, 63, 105, 137, 154, 166, 169, 175, 176, 177, 184
immune, 24, 36, 170, 171
immunological, 25
in vitro fertilization, 146
incentive, 22, 29, 49, 76, 78, 79, 81, 109, 149, 165, 192

information, 26, 27, 48, 122, 124, 141, 150, 152, 153, 154, 159, 161, 164-5, 169, 182, 184, 187, 189, 192, 195
innovation, 14, 22, 85, 89, 119, 169, 175, 181, 183, 187, 188, 190-3, 195
innovative, 11, 17, 51, 154, 156, 188
innovators, 13, 154, 169, 184, 187, 191
instantaneous gratification, 96
interactive video, 167
isolation, 162, 166
Japanese, 14, 36, 81, 169, 175, 188, 191
kidney stones, 90, 177
laser, 150, 174, 177, 178, 188
LDL-cholesterol, 130
life extension, 184
lifestyle, 122, 125
listen to patient, 154
litigation, 21, 112, 117, 160
longevity, 32, 125, 147
Lord Beveridge, 29, 46

malpractice, 21
managed care, 150, 151
market forces, 74, 75, 147, 183, 184
marketing, 17, 155, 165
media, 14, 19, 26, 30, 34, 73, 118, 123, 133, 152
medical computing, 155, 157, 192
Medical Research Council (MRC), 115, 192
medical mind-net, 166
medical history/record, 140, 141, 157, 192
medical-industrial, 17, 30
Medicare, 13, 25, 29, 37, 38, 49, 52, 84, 113, 126, 150, 154, 175, 184, 190, 193
mediocre, 188
memory, 140
mental/emotional illness, 131, 142, 144
modem, 35
molecular biology, 28, 183
monitor, 84, 87, 106, 113, 138, 141, 142, 143, 144, 148, 158, 173
morale, 11, 13, 21, 111, 114, 195
motivate, 22, 65, 76, 81, 122, 148
MRI, 21
National Health Service (NHS), 29, 44, 65
National Institutes of Health (NIH), 53, 192
negation rate, 98, 99, 102

neurodegenerative, 25, 131
New Economy, 11, 27, 30, 90, 93, 169
New Brunswick, 111
Newfoundland, 111, 161
nurse practitioner, 101
Ontario, 38, 57, 60, 72, 75, 86, 89, 92, 97, 112, 130, 135, 137 146, 156, 168, 184, 190, 191, 192, 193
Ontario Medical Association (OMA), 102, 103, 104, 115, 130
optical card, 139
Oregon, 40, 134, 185
osteoarthritis, 132
outcomes, 68, 112, 113, 138, 156, 195
over-the-counter drugs, 141
overutilizing, 16, 52
paradigm, 22, 23, 26, 27, 28, 48, 64, 85, 109, 120, 134, 153, 181, 182, 193, 195
Parkinson's disease, 145
patient expectations, 21, 34
patient demand, 22
peptides, 172
pharmaceutical, 25, 47, 163, 170, 174, 179, 182, 188
pharmacy, 68
photodynamic therapy, 178
placebo, 23, 24, 52, 57, 117, 148
plaque, 128, 130, 137,
prescriptions, 20, 30, 68, 77, 87, 99, 141
preventive, 20, 26, 49, 69, 73, 101, 106, 107, 112, 118, 121-2, 124, 126, 131, 136-7, 153-5, 183-4
primary care, 19, 96, 106
private sector, 57, 90, 105, 142, 156, 159, 176, 183, 191, 192
privatization, 105, 133, 137, 185
procedure-oriented, 114
prostate cancer, 146
psychiatrists, 144
quality of life, 127, 153, 184
quality assurance, 54, 150, 156, 182, 187, 189
Quebec, 107, 109, 111, 139, 140, 159
rational drug design, 172
rationing, 17, 37, 40, 46, 73
reassurance, 148
reassure, 26
receptor chemistry, 172

recombinant DNA, 32, 171
reform, 13, 147, 184
reinvent, 11, 14, 188
reversing CAD, 128, 136
risk factors, 72, 125, 129, 136, 165
roster, 98, 99, 102
Royal Commission, 14, 37, 83, 134, 146, 149
salary, 14, 28, 51, 97, 106, 108, 113, 120, 145, 183, 195
Saskatchewan, 74
screening, 26, 122, 124, 126, 127, 129, 130, 175, 177
secondary, 65
self-care, 143, 144, 173
self-help, 35, 123
seniors, 36, 38, 91, 139
senstatin, 32
serious illness, 62
severence package, 78
sick notes, 80
silent cardiovascular disease, 128
silicone breast implant, 57, 70, 91, 150
simulation, 174
smart drugs, 33
Smartcard, 68, 138, 139, 143, 157
socialism, 181
software, 68, 158, 194
specialist, 15, 19, 96, 108, 114, 159, 180
spinal cord injuries, 59
SRTC/ SR&ED), 193
stakeholders, 15, 162, 193
standards, 189
strategic plan, 156, 187, 188, 189, 192
stratify risk, 129
stroke, 20, 32
Swedish, 74, 79, 90
Switzerland, 22, 23
talk to patient, 154
telecommunications, 11, 30, 35, 61, 155, 159, 162, 169
television, 19, 30, 31, 122, 136, 151
tertiary, 62
tests, 20, 26, 63, 65, 105, 117, 122-3, 126-8, 136-8, 143, 147-9, 152
The Globe and Mail, 68, 76, 77, 81, 84, 89, 92, 117, 135
The Financial Post, 68

tools, 21, 38, 68, 79, 107, 112, 124, 154, 157, 168, 174, 175, 178
Toronto Star, 74, 91, 191
underserviced, 15, 107, 112
unrealistic, 30
user fees, 38, 70, 74, 109

virtual reality, 186
vision, 187
visualization, 154, 158, 174, 176, 186
voice-entry, 141

walk-in clinic, 16, 88, 96, 113, 144
waste, 16,19- 20, 22, 38, 57, 81, 118, 130, 135, 146, 148, 149, 151, 184, 187, 189, 194
wellness, 49, 73, 102, 125, 165, 183
wish fulfillment, 153
worried well, 148, 149

zero tolerance, 35, 179